your
12-WEEK
to running guide

FROM YOUR ARMCHAIR TO A 5 KM RACE IN 12 WEEKS

Fact box sources (note: conversions are from g to oz (US) and from ml to fl oz (US). (1) UK Department of Health. (2) USGS. (3) UK Department of Health. (4) UK Department of Health: Sport and Exercise Medicine: a Fresh Approach (2012). (5) McDonald's, Pizza Hut, KFC (all US). (6) P Lally, European Journal of Social Psychology. (7) US National Health Interview Survey (2010). (8) Harvard Heart Letter (July 2004). (9) Coca-Cola (US), Starbucks (US). (10) UK Department of Health: Start Active, Stay Active (2011) and US The President's Council on Physical Fitness and Sport. (11) UK Department of Health: Start Active, Stay Active (2011) and www.bootsdiets.com. (12) US National Sleep Foundation. (13) UK NHS Sport and Exercise Medicine: A Fresh Approach (2011). (14) US The President's Council on Physical Fitness and Sports: Fast Facts About Sports Nutrition. (15) Drinkaware.co.uk. (16) US The President's Council on Physical Fitness and Sports: Fast Facts About Sports Nutrition. (17) US The President's Council on Physical Fitness and Sports: Exercise and Weight Control. (18) AM Williamson and AM Feyer, British Medical Journal (2000). (19) USGS. (20) Fitness Australia. (21) *Triathlon: Serious About Your Sport* (NHP). (22) Olaf Lahl et al, University of Dusseldorf (2008). (23) JH Stubbe et al, The association between exercise participation and well-being (2006) and various others. Photos: iStockphoto.com and www.sxc.hu, P4-5 Said-w. P15 Ariel da Silva Parreira. P35 John Nyberg, www.hdrfoto.dk. P62 Jesper Markward Olsen, jmolsen.

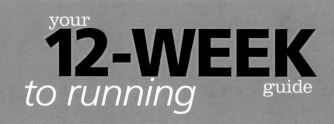

your 12-WEEK guide to running

FROM YOUR ARMCHAIR TO A 5 KM RACE IN 12 WEEKS

by Daniel Ford

Training programme by Paul Cowcher

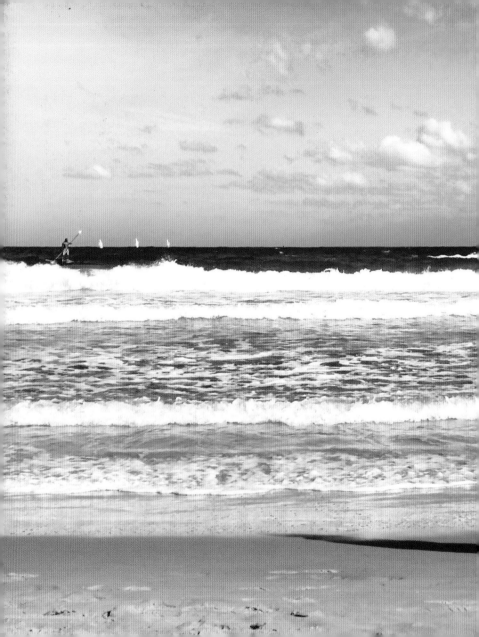

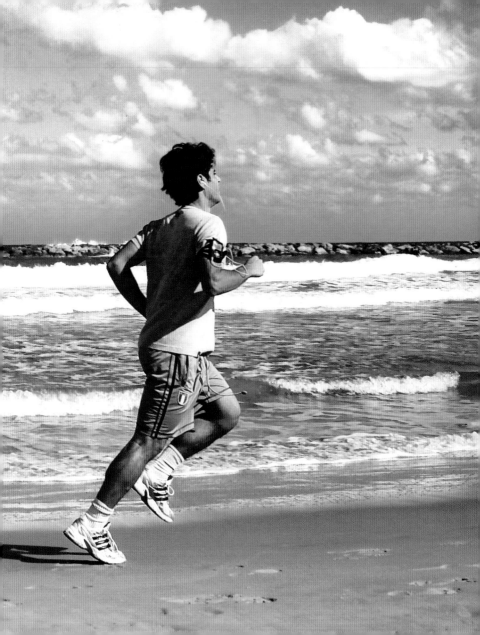

your
12-WEEK plan

2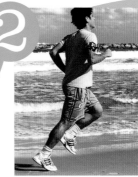

1
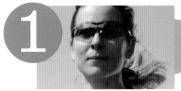

Making the commitment
An important step is simply deciding to go for it…

Get running
Now it's time to get moving. Slowly and gently at first, nothing too much to start with…

8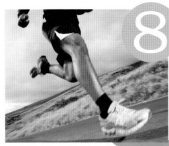

7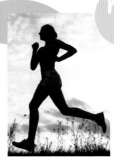

You're halfway there
Time to take stock. Think how far you've come in a short time…

Recommit and look forward
Remind yourself why you started running and look ahead to the finish…

10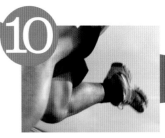

9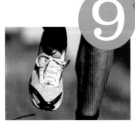

Now push on
It's time to crank up the energy levels…

Cruise control
You're feeling fit and healthy. This running is becoming a stroll in the park…

3

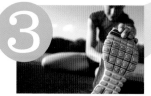

Stretch out and relax

The importance of rest days, sleep and stretching…

4

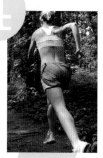

Make exercise a habit

Suddenly running is a regular part of your routine…

6

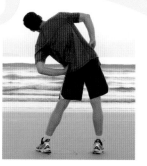

Feel the benefits

You will already be starting to feel better and fitter. This is what you've been working for…

5

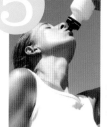

In the groove

Running should be feeling easier and smoother. Enjoy the rhythm of it…

11

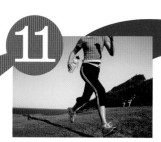

You're nearly there

It's time to start winding down and concentrate on the race…

12

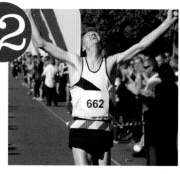

It's race week

This is what you've been aiming for. You're ready to run 5 km…

introduction

Welcome, your 12-week challenge starts here...

You have already taken the first important step towards completing this challenge, from your armchair to a 5 km race in 12 weeks, because you have seen this book online or in a bookshop and thought to yourself, "This is what I need; this is for me." The best way to use this book is to view the next 12 weeks as a series of small steps. Add them all up and you will complete the end goal. And because you are reading this you have already completed the first, and probably the most important step of all. Hey, aren't these steps easy?

Think of it this way: you don't host a successful dinner party by worrying about the final result and deciding that there is no way you can get all the food and drink together and still welcome your guests with a smile on your face. You simply picture the end result – plates piled high with your delicious food and happy faces supping away – and set about all the small tasks needed to get to that end result. You know it won't happen with a simple click of the fingers (getting from your armchair to a 5 km race won't either) so you just concentrate on the small tasks such as marinating the meat, chopping the vegetables, setting the table and so on, because you

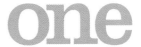

There is only one thing you should be concentrating on right now and that is to start exercising. Don't attempt to give up smoking and drinking and start eating salads just yet. You are more likely to give up if you try to change too much at once.

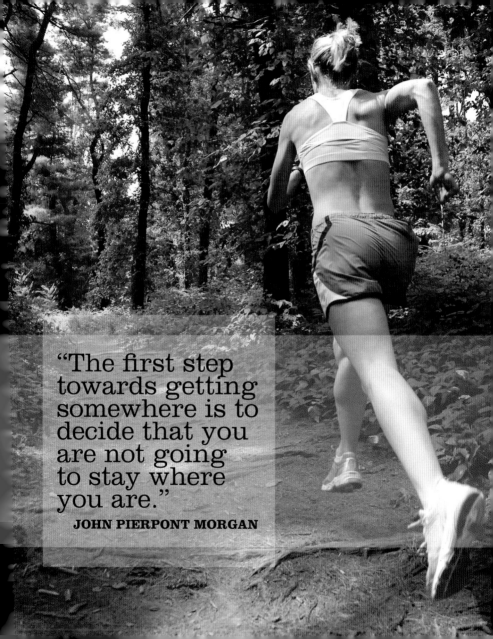

"The first step towards getting somewhere is to decide that you are not going to stay where you are."

JOHN PIERPONT MORGAN

know all the small tasks will eventually add up to the end result you have pictured in your mind.

Different people will have different reasons for doing this challenge. Maybe you want to lose a bit of weight? Get into a dress that's got a bit too tight? Encourage yourself to eat healthier? Feel more energized during the day? Or maybe it was a bet with a friend in the pub who teased you that your sporting days were behind you? All of these are perfectly fine, and are common motivators, but remember the goal is to get out of your armchair and finish a 5 km race. Do not obsess with the other things like weight loss, your diet or losing your bet; these are by-products of what you are doing and will look after themselves.

It's unlikely, but not impossible, that you cross the line in 12 weeks weighing the same as you do right now, or that you somehow complete the race fuelled on your current diet of pizza and chicken wings. Things take time, every person is different and there are many other factors involved. If you stress that the weight is not falling off after a couple of jogs around the park or that the pizza delivery man still knows you by your first name during these 12 weeks then the only result will be a loss of motivation and you'll be back where you started – in your armchair.

So the next step is to take a few seconds right now to visualize the end result. Close your eyes if it helps.

hear

Listen to your body. You know when you are feeling good and you know when you are not because your body tells you. Follow the programme and listen to advice but always remember the best guide you will have is your own body.

see

Make sure you visualize your success before you have even taken a physical step towards it. Your mind and body work together as a team and your head is the leader so take time to picture your success right away.

It doesn't matter if you are on a train, at home, wherever, or if you think this visualization stuff is all a load of old nonsense (most of us think the same) just take a few moments to see the end result.

This is all about seeing yourself in 12 weeks' time bounding across the finish line feeling good with a smile on your face. Picture a few of the details like the sun on your face and the applause from your partner or friends as you finish the challenge. Oh, go on then, you can imagine yourself slimmer and sexier as well…

Oi, you two at the back who have skipped this bit! Come on, picture your success… That's better.

How to use your book

Right, now you've pictured the end result in your mind it's time to start taking the steps needed to get there. You won't need to be a rocket scientist to realize that this book is broken down into 12 large steps. Each will include a brief overview of what the focus of that particular week is all about. Read this at the end of the previous week so you've got time to digest it. As with above, visualize the success of the week (come on, you're an old hand at this). Don't skip these few seconds of visualization as they are important in firming up the week ahead in your mind. You will also find snippets of information on things such as food and drink, mental fitness, sleep, and so on, that you can use during your 12 weeks.

The most important page in each section is Your Training Programme and Diary. Again, look over this page at the end of the previous week so the information has plenty of time to sink in. Also ensure you make space in your diary for each day's activity and don't relegate them to, "I'll fit that in somewhere," or you'll get to the end of the day and realize there is no time left. Treat each session as you would an important meeting at work or an appointment with your child's school.

At the bottom of these pages you will also see some traffic lights offering a 'Do This', 'Consider This' and a 'Don't Do This'. These are small tips that you can take on board during the week if you wish. You will also see a 'Reward' on this page, a little something to look forward to when the week is completed. Thoughtful eh? Ah, it's nothing. Use the small notes column to the right of each day to record how you're feeling. It's a great way to end a session and fun to look back on later. You will be amazed at how quickly you progress.

Finally, at the end of each chapter there is a summary of what you have achieved that week. Again, use the notes column to jot down your thoughts and feelings as this will help draw a line under the week and help prepare you for the next one. Then it's time for you to give yourself a pat on the back and refer back to your reward.

when

When thinking of taking up an exercise programme for the first time or after an extended break it's important that you check with your doctor that you are fit and healthy enough. Explain your plan and get the thumbs up before starting.

Your aim this week

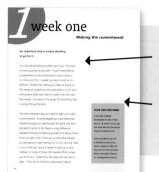

At the end of each week read what's in store for the coming week so you have time to digest it.

This is where you will find a snapshot of your aim for the week. Elsewhere in the section you will find small snippets of information on things such as food and drink or mental fitness.

Training programme

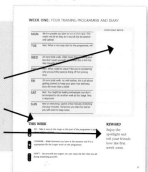

Make sure you diarize your sessions as if they are important appointments. They are.

Jot down your thoughts even if it's just, "Saw Mrs Smith as I set off for my run. She looked impressed!" or "Felt great today".

These are additional tips you can use during your week.

This is what you are looking forward to at the end of the week.

What you have achieved

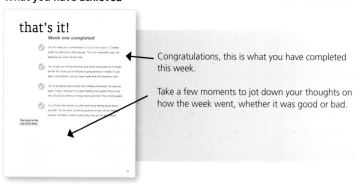

Congratulations, this is what you have completed this week.

Take a few moments to jot down your thoughts on how the week went, whether it was good or bad.

1 week one

Making the commitment

An important step is simply deciding to go for it...

You should be feeling excited right now. The start of every journey brings with it that mixed feeling of apprehension and anticipation about what is to come and this 12-week journey should be no different. Bottle that feeling you have of being on the verge of something new and whip it out if your enthusiasm levels ever start to wane over the next few weeks. You *are* on the verge of something new so enjoy the excitement.

The next important step you need to take is to make a commitment. To some degree you have done that already because you have bought the book and have decided to go for it. But there is a big difference between thinking something yourself and telling others what you plan to do. Once you've told other people you are about to start training for a 5 km race the 'idea is out of the bag' and it is harder to give up or stop halfway. So none of those half-hearted efforts where you think you, "Might try a few days and see how it goes". That sort of thinking is doomed to failure.

YOUR AIM THIS WEEK

Is to make a public declaration to run a 5 km race in 12 weeks. Go on, get out there and tell the world what you intend to do.

You've decided to go for it already so now is the time to share it. After all, once you've told everyone about your plans there is no turning back is there?

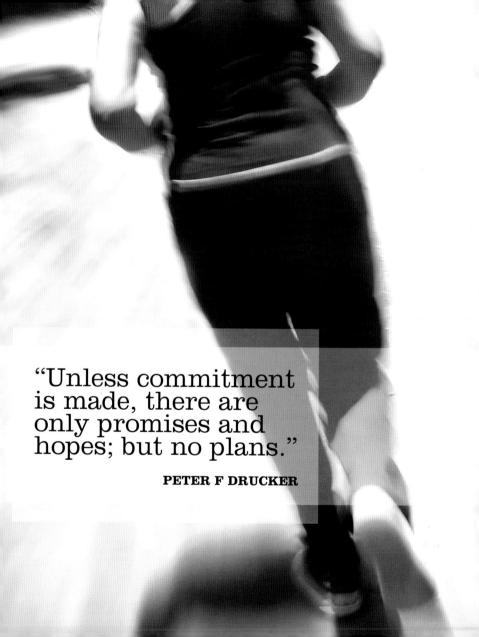

"Unless commitment is made, there are only promises and hopes; but no plans."

PETER F DRUCKER

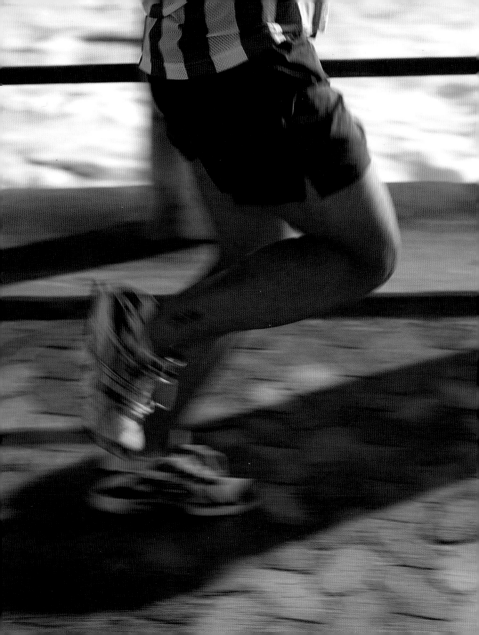

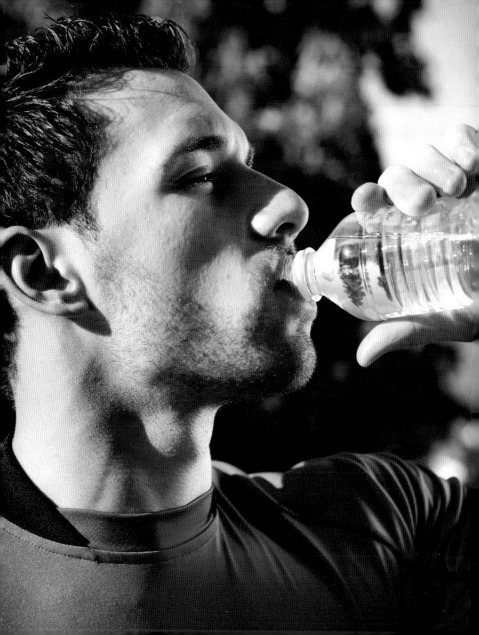

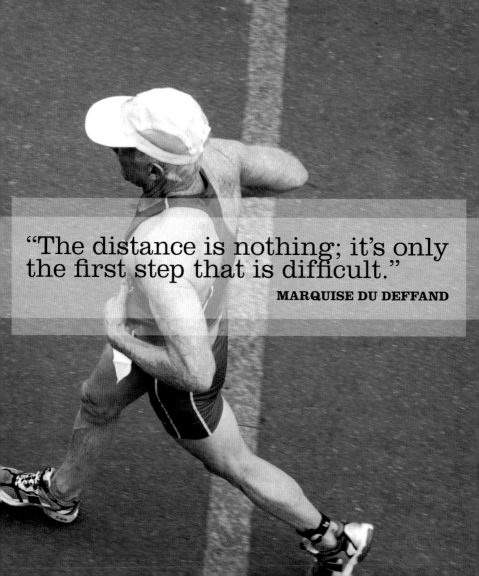

"The distance is nothing; it's only the first step that is difficult."

MARQUISE DU DEFFAND

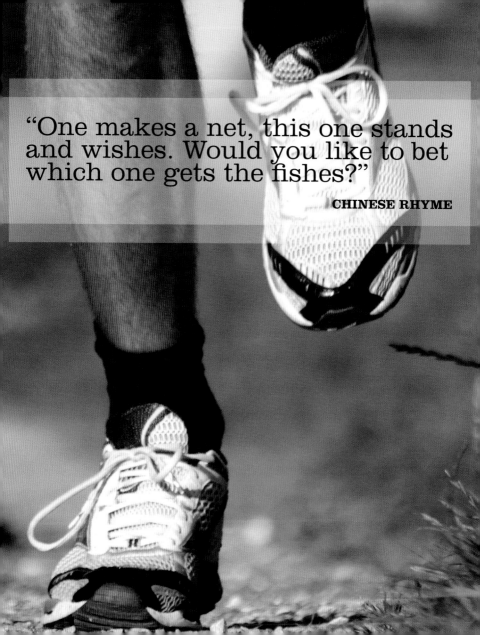

"One makes a net, this one stands and wishes. Would you like to bet which one gets the fishes?"

CHINESE RHYME

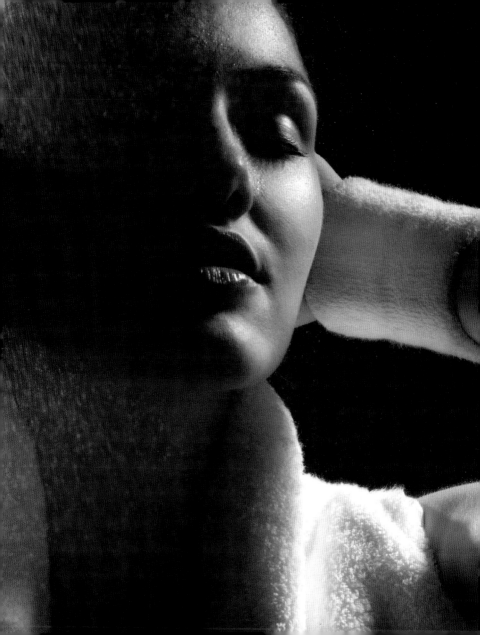

Women doing enough exercise

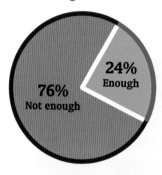

24% **Enough**

76% **Not enough**

Only 24 per cent of women (37 per cent of men) in the UK do enough exercise according to government health guidelines. Well done, you are on your way to joining the minority!

The figures show just how easy it is for most people to fall into the trap of not keeping fit. Remind yourself of this if you ever feel like giving up in the coming weeks. (1)

do this in secret but people who share their plans out loud are much more likely to follow them through to the end, which is due to a mixture of wanting to display success to others and a fear of being viewed as a failure. Smokers who tell friends they are giving up display determination and are much more likely to succeed than those who don't and it's the same with anything else, including this 12-week programme.

So day one is simple enough, if a little daunting for some. The rest of the week is really all about shaking off those exercise cobwebs with a few very short walks and stretches. You may feel you're fit enough or be excited enough to hit the road straight away; after all walks are for old people with dogs right? But stick to it. Don't worry, you've got 12 weeks and plenty of time to sprint past your neighbour's house with a grin on your face.

Just use this first week as a way of getting moving again with 'planned' exercise. You probably do a fair bit of walking in your daily life already – to the shops, the bus stop, down the pub and so on – but these are all ad hoc activities. Informal exercise like this is important, and will even be incorporated into the next 12 weeks, but having a session planned, even a walk, means you will be less likely to miss it. You will also get that buzz from having 'done something'.

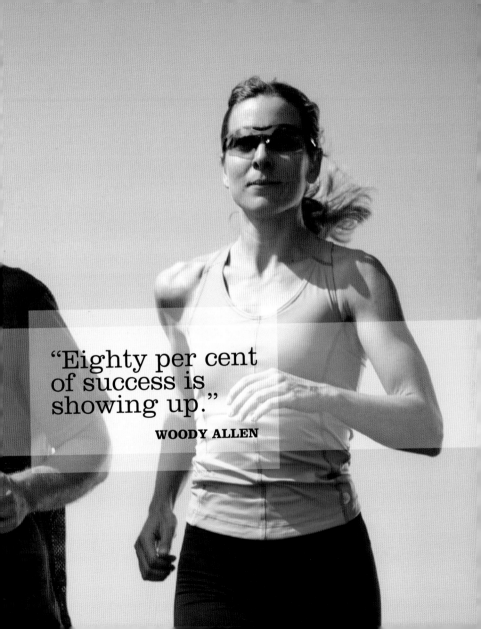

"Eighty per cent of success is showing up."

WOODY ALLEN

that's it!

Week one completed

✓ You've made your commitment to run a 5 km race in 12 weeks public by telling five other people. This is an important step. No keeping your plans secret now!

✓ You've got out of that armchair and done some exercise. It might be the first time you've followed a programme or maybe it's just been a long break, but you have made that all-important start.

✓ You've probably rediscovered that child-like enthusiasm for exercise again. Enjoy it because it's a great feeling and a great thing to tap into should you feel your energy levels waning in the coming weeks.

✓ You should have woken up after exercising feeling good about yourself. You've done something positive so you will be feeling positive mentally as well as physically now you've got started.

Your notes at the
end of the week

23

2 week two

Now is the time to start running

Okay, let's get moving. Slowly and gently at first, nothing too much to start with…

Up until now everything has been about getting your mind ready for the weeks ahead and getting used to setting aside some time for exercise. Now it's time to get going. There will still be a lot of walking and even some cross-training sessions of other sports (like swimming or cycling) worked in later on to keep boredom at bay but now it's time get moving.

There are a few things to consider when you start running again after a break of months or years. Firstly there is no shame in stopping to walk every so often at the beginning. In fact, run-walk, using alternate periods of running interspersed with walks is a perfectly accepted practice in the running world, and has even been used successfully by some top runners. You will notice that the programme includes alternate periods of walking and running (more walking than running to start with). This is a good training technique even if you can't get it out of your head that stopping to walk is 'cheating'.

YOUR AIM THIS WEEK

Is to accept that you should not do more than the programme sets out – even if your enthusiasm is sky high at the moment.

The best way to reach your end goal is to slowly build your fitness and confidence. People who do too much at the start are often nowhere to be seen at the end.

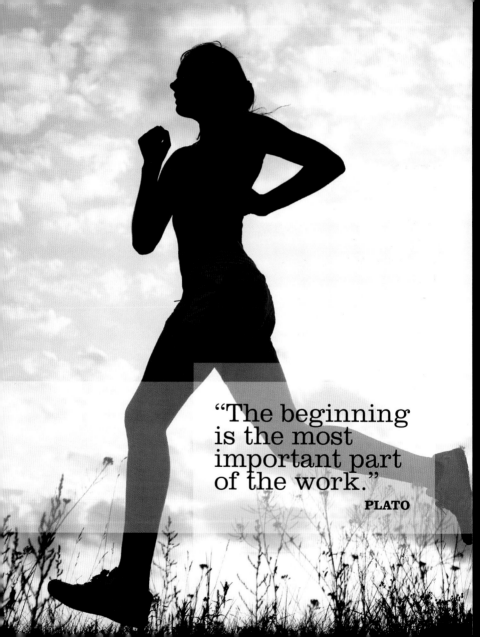

"The beginning is the most important part of the work."

PLATO

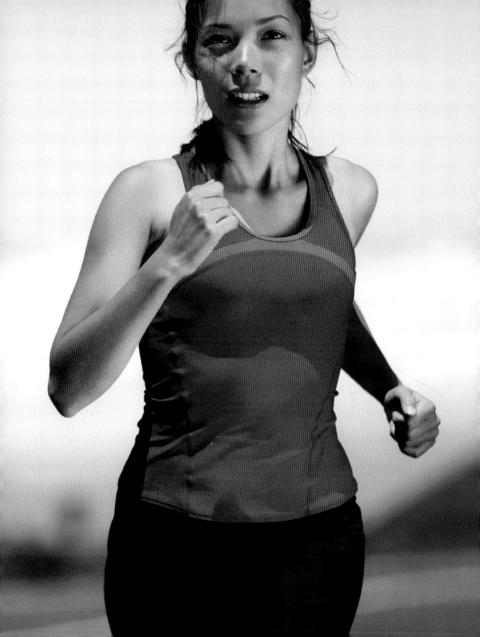

WEEK TWO: YOUR TRAINING PROGRAMME AND DIARY

		YOUR DAILY NOTES
MON	9 mins brisk walk, 1 min jog, repeat x3 (total 30 mins). The short jogs are all about getting you moving so keep it easy.	
TUE	Rest. Enjoy a day off.	
WED	5 mins walk, 3 mins jog, 5 mins brisk walk (total 13 mins). Don't be tempted to push yourself on the jog.	
THU	Rest. Consider a bit of stretching when you get the opportunity, but make sure your muscles are warm first.	
FRI	9 mins brisk walk, 1 min jog, repeat x3 (total 30 mins). Try to stay loose and relaxed when it comes to the short jogs.	
SAT	Rest.	
SUN	Rest or stretching. Stretching is as much to get loose for the next day as it is to ease the muscles from the exercise you have already done.	

THIS WEEK

 DO – Plan your week in advance to make sure you know what days and time you will be training.

 CONSIDER – Increasing the amount of water you drink. Try to have two extra glasses every day.

 DON'T – Panic if you miss a day's training because the programme is flexible and you can switch rest and training days around if you have to.

REWARD

Enjoy your favourite meal – curry, burger and fries, whatever – without guilt or worry.

Think of how small children run: they sprint flat out until they are exhausted, put hands on hips to get some air and off they go again. We are not suggesting you adopt the same 'flat out' approach but stop-start exercise of that style is an excellent way to build your fitness. So rid yourself of the worry about the odd walk. That's not to say you use this as an excuse, by the way. Instead keep your mind on the end goal (5 km) and don't worry about the process of getting there.

There is also the problem of starting off too fast when running. Maybe it's because we remember our running prowess at school that we all still believe we can just pull on some shorts and head up the road as if nothing has changed. Start slower than you think you should, especially on your first few runs, then slow down some more. Don't worry if you feel as if the snails in your neighbour's garden are catching you up; you've got 12 weeks. A good rule-of-thumb way to check you are going at the right pace is to see if you can hold a conversation when running: if you can't ease up a bit.

Which leads us on to the dreaded worry of people watching you run, or worse still, actually seeing someone you know when out exercising. Do I look silly when I run? Does my excess weight still show despite that baggy top I chose? If that's you, then assuming where you choose to run is safe, you'll have to use the early mornings and late nights when no one is about and you will feel less self-conscious.

2.4litres

Every day you need to replace 2.4 litres (five pints) of water that is lost or expelled from your body. Although some will come from the food you eat it's important that you drink plenty of water during the day to ensure you do not become dehydrated. (2)

Choose at least five friends, family or colleagues who you will tell about your plan to run 5 km. Don't become an instant office bore by bursting in wearing your new fitness clothing and carrying a healthy snack for lunch (although feel free to wave this fine book around, of course). Simply wait for the right time and slip it into the conversation.

"What did I do this weekend? Oh, I bought a new book and have decided to train for a 5 km race." "What am I doing this week? Well, I am about to start training for a 5 km race." That sort of thing.

Be prepared for a mixed response, especially when your news spreads on the gossip grapevine. Some people will congratulate you, others will raise their eyebrows and certain people may even laugh. Don't let this put you off one bit; in fact use these responses to spur you on this week. Pick at least one person who you feel sure will encourage you in your plans but don't avoid those who may give you negative feedback – that usually comes because those people are jealous they are not doing it or fearful they couldn't do it.

To some of you this will sound worse than actually starting the training itself but that's exactly why you need to do it. Of course, if you absolutely cannot face telling another soul then it shouldn't mean you should stop right now. It is possible to

50

Is the number of minutes you will be exercising this week. This is probably less than the time you might spend having a coffee with a friend or even watching your favourite television programme. Not a lot when you think of it like that is it? Make sure you find the time for exercise just as you would any other activity.

		YOUR DAILY NOTES
MON	Tell five people you plan to run a 5 km race. This might not be as easy as it sounds but be positive and upbeat.	
TUE	Rest. What a nice easy start to the programme, eh?	
WED	20 mins brisk walk. Walk faster than strolling pace but don't push yourself; remember this is the first step towards 5 km.	
THU	Rest. What could be easier? Bet you're wondering why you put this exercise thing off for so long now.	
FRI	30 mins brisk walk. As with before, this is all about getting started so keep your pace nice and easy, but a bit more than a stroll.	
SAT	Rest. You might be feeling enthusiastic but don't be tempted to do another walk at this stage. Rest is important.	
SUN	Rest or stretching. Spend a few minutes stretching out your muscles. Tomorrow you start for real so you will want to keep loose.	

THIS WEEK

 DO – Take it easy at this stage as this part of the programme is just about getting started.

 CONSIDER – What footwear you have at the moment and if it is appropriate for the longer work on the programme.

 DON'T – Set yourself any targets yet, just enjoy the fact that you are doing something positive.

REWARD

Enjoy the spotlight and tell your friends how the first week went.

Or better still, don't care what anyone thinks, as this is about you anyway.

Whatever you do, just try to enjoy the fact that you are out of that armchair and exercising. Your body is doing something again other than slouching in a chair, even if it is for only a few minutes at a time right now. You'll huff and puff at first ("How did I get this unfit?") and even turn a darker shade of beetroot, but console yourself that this is the normal process of getting fit. Needless to say, if you feel at any stage you've done too much, stop and take a breather or stop altogether. The training programme has been carefully worked out, but only you can truly know how much you can manage, so don't overdo it.

On the flip side, do not be tempted to do more than what is in the programme even if you are feeling like Wonder Woman or Superman. The programme has been designed for a gradual progression towards the end goal and to make sure you avoid injury. Some of the keenest people do too much at the start of an exercise programme but they are not there at the end because they have burnt up all their enthusiasm.

You will be amazed at how quickly you start to improve so remember the huffing and puffing because it won't last long. You will probably experience some stiffness in your legs this week so remember to stretch out your muscles so they are ready for the next run.

Daily calorie intake

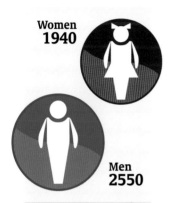

Women
1940

Men
2550

There is no need to get calorie obsessed but nutritional values are clearly marked on most food we buy so it's easy enough to keep an eye on your intake.

What you need per day depends on various factors such as your height, weight and your lifestyle. The chart shows the estimated averages by UK authorities. (3)

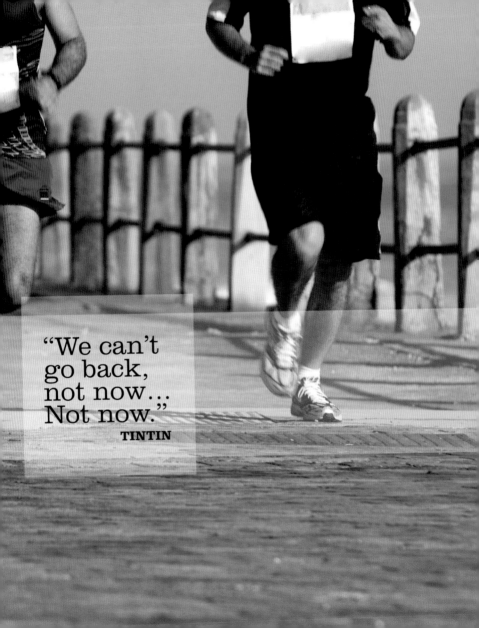

"We can't
go back,
not now...
Not now."

TINTIN

that's it!

Week two completed

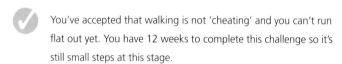 You've accepted that walking is not 'cheating' and you can't run flat out yet. You have 12 weeks to complete this challenge so it's still small steps at this stage.

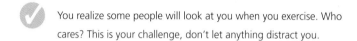 You realize some people will look at you when you exercise. Who cares? This is your challenge, don't let anything distract you.

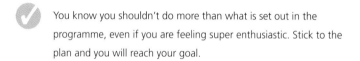 You know you shouldn't do more than what is set out in the programme, even if you are feeling super enthusiastic. Stick to the plan and you will reach your goal.

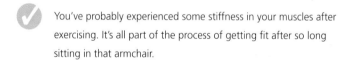 You've probably experienced some stiffness in your muscles after exercising. It's all part of the process of getting fit after so long sitting in that armchair.

Your notes at the
end of the week

3 week three

Stretch out and relax

The importance of rest days, good sleep and lots of stretching…

If we were to tell you that the most important days in the programme are the rest days would that cheer you up? Thought so. When you exercise you put your body under stress. It's the good stress that pushes your muscles beyond what they are normally used to (but within their limits) not the bad stress you get from your boss at work or the rude person behind the till in the supermarket.

And because you have pushed your body outside of its normal parameters it needs to recover and rebuild. That's where rest days come in. Push, rebuild, push, rebuild. Think of it as slowly putting together a series of building blocks in your body until you are ready for the end goal: a 5 km race. You exercise to push your body to make it stronger and fitter, then you let it recover and rebuild so it is ready for the next stage. That's why any fitness programme should be gradual, because it is indeed putting those blocks together bit by bit. So always remember that the rest days are important. That doesn't mean you have to lie

YOUR AIM THIS WEEK

Is to understand the importance of rest days. Now rest can't be difficult can it? Rest days are when your body recovers and rebuilds after exercise so treat them with respect.

You also need to be trying to get a good sleep and to be getting into the habit of stretching out your muscles before and after exercise.

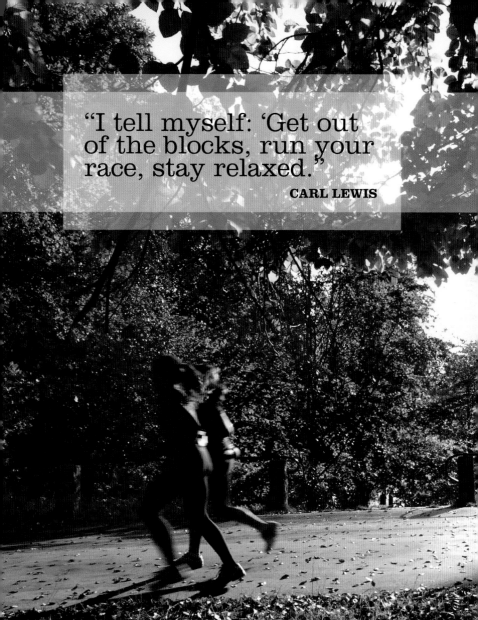

"I tell myself: 'Get out of the blocks, run your race, stay relaxed.'"

CARL LEWIS

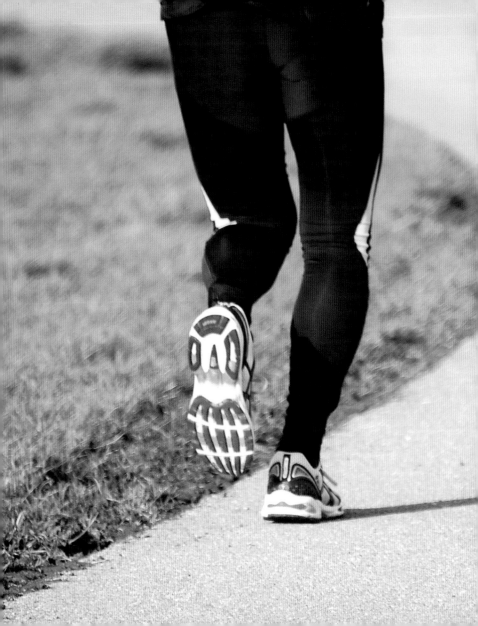

WEEK THREE: YOUR TRAINING PROGRAMME AND DIARY

		YOUR DAILY NOTES
MON	8 mins brisk walk, 2 mins jog, repeat x3 (total 30 mins). The jogging will slowly increase but the bulk of work is still at a brisk walking pace.	
TUE	Rest.	
WED	5 mins walk, 5 mins jog, 5 mins brisk walk (total 15 mins). This is a good workout that takes less time than it would to make and drink a coffee.	
THU	Rest. Hopefully you are now getting into the habit of stretching on your rest days, even if it is just for a few minutes.	
FRI	8 mins brisk walk, 2 mins jog, repeat x3 (total 30 mins).	
SAT	Rest. Enjoy a nice, relaxing weekend.	
SUN	Rest or stretching. Remember to look ahead and schedule your training days by putting them into your phone or diary.	

THIS WEEK

 DO – Start thinking about your posture while exercising. A good posture will keep those aches and pains away.

 CONSIDER – Joining in group exercises, or finding an exercise partner. It is a lot easier to train with other people.

 DON'T – Don't push yourself too hard while exercising or you will find yourself straining.

REWARD

Book yourself a relaxing body massage.

prone on the couch from morning till night, because you still have a life to lead, but it does mean you shouldn't do an extra session just because you are feeling enthusiastic on those days. If you do you will feel jaded when you return to the programme and more likely to pack it in altogether.

If resting is important then it stands to reason that sleep is very important. When you exercise, especially at the beginning, your body is likely to want more sleep (to help it recover and rebuild). Only you will know the extent of this but try to get in a bit of extra sleep if you can. A regular sleep pattern also helps ('catching up' on your sleep on the weekend is not the best thing). Of course, here in the real world it's not always possible to get more sleep and keep it regular. However, within the confines of your lifestyle, try to make a concerted effort to get the best sleep you possibly can.

In addition to sleep there are many other things you can to do to help you relax, such as listening to music, taking a hot bath or watching films and sports recordings for inspiration and motivation.

Now on to stretching. A lot of people skip stretching because they think it looks silly (well, it does, we are with you on that). All that bending over, grunting, and struggling to get your leg up on a bench. But remember that stretching is very important

38%

Unless you're a particular fan of hospital food, being inactive doesn't really hold much appeal. UK research has found that inactive people spend 38 per cent more days in hospital than active people, visit their doctor 5.5 per cent more and use specialist services 13 per cent more. (4)

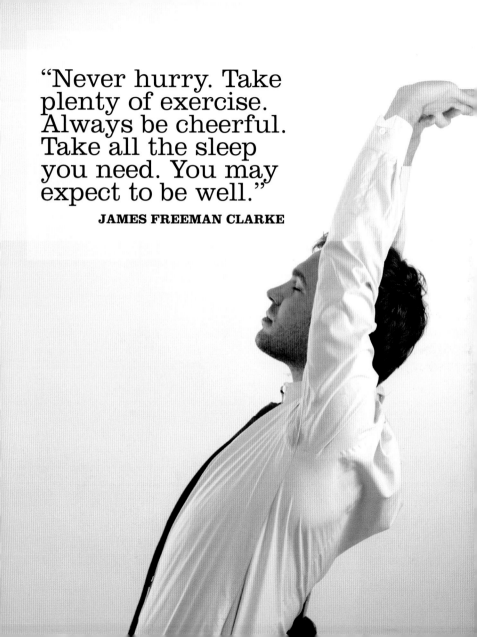

"Never hurry. Take plenty of exercise. Always be cheerful. Take all the sleep you need. You may expect to be well."

JAMES FREEMAN CLARKE

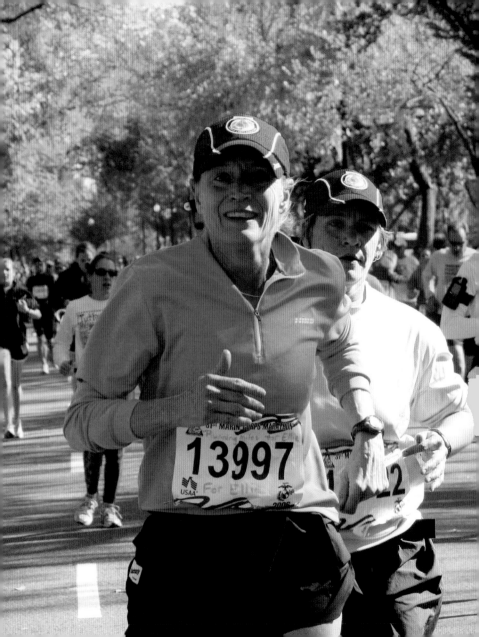

when you are exercising. In fact, it's important for everyone, but it is especially important for you now because every time you work your muscles they tighten and contract (that's partly where stiffness comes from).

Calories in takeaways

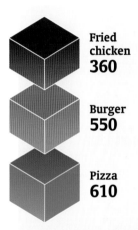

Fried chicken
360

Burger
550

Pizza
610

Nothing beats a tasty takeaway, but keep an eye on the calories. The chart above refers to a Big Mac (215 g, 7.6 oz), a Pizza Hut Pepperoni 6-inch (15 cm) Personal Pan Pizza, a KFC chicken breast (163 g, 5.8 oz). (5)

So get into the habit of stretching before you exercise (stretch very gently as your muscles will not be warm) but also after you have exercised. The after bit is easy to skip, we understand, because at the end of the session all you want is a drink and a sit down. Don't be tempted, though, because, if anything, it is more important to stretch after a session than before it. Your muscles will be warm and more receptive to being worked. A few minutes stretching the back of your legs (calves, hamstrings, glutes), the front of your legs (quads), your back, shoulders and neck will have you feeling loose and refreshed as well as help you to avoid injury.

Stretching is the one thing that we would encourage you to do on the rest days in the programme. Again, just a few minutes on these days will help keep your muscles relaxed and they will be better prepared for the next session. Even if you are pushed for time (who isn't?) there are always spare moments in the day when you can stretch out your muscles, whether it's a calf stretch in the shower in the morning or a gentle hamstring stretch or neck roll as you sit at your desk at work.

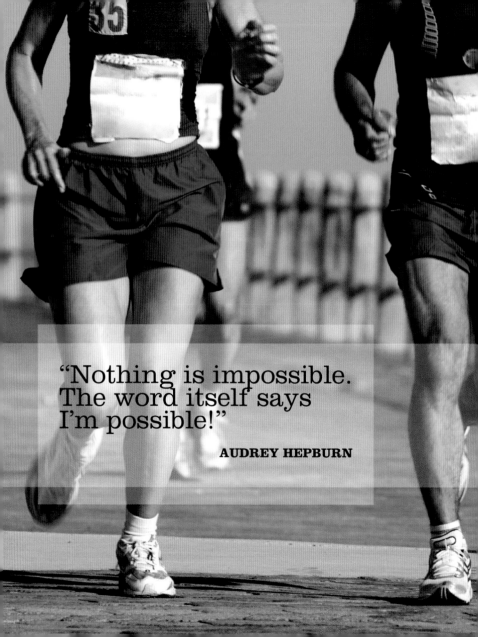

"Nothing is impossible.
The word itself says
I'm possible!"

AUDREY HEPBURN

that's it!

Week three completed

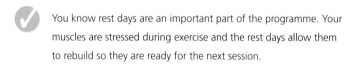 You know rest days are an important part of the programme. Your muscles are stressed during exercise and the rest days allow them to rebuild so they are ready for the next session.

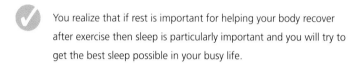 You realize that if rest is important for helping your body recover after exercise then sleep is particularly important and you will try to get the best sleep possible in your busy life.

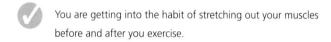 You are getting into the habit of stretching out your muscles before and after you exercise.

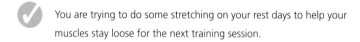 You are trying to do some stretching on your rest days to help your muscles stay loose for the next training session.

Your notes at the end of the week

week four

Make exercising a habit

Suddenly running is a regular part of your routine…

If you do something regularly enough then it will become a habit. Chances are you didn't sit down one day and decide it would be a good idea to spend your evenings running around after your children, or slumped in front of the television with a takeaway every night so that you got to bed feeling as if you've had no time to yourself. Time, or the lack of it, simply got the better of you and you repeated it enough so that it became a habit.

But just as things you don't particularly want can become habits in your life so can things that you do want. If you've stuck to the programme so far and are still reading this then it's fair to assume you want exercising to become a habit (at least until the 12 weeks is up and you've run that 5 km).

As you are still only a couple of weeks down the line the chances are that training is still a novelty and it hasn't become a habit yet. All you need to do at this stage is stick at it and before you know it your

YOUR AIM THIS WEEK

Is to keep going, knowing that by doing so you are making exercise a habit in your life.

Good habits, the same as bad habits, are created simply by repeating the same action. Before you know it you will be pulling on your training gear as if it is second nature.

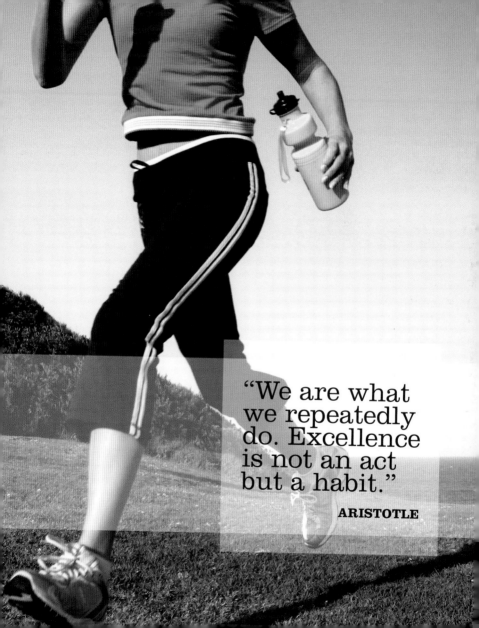

"We are what we repeatedly do. Excellence is not an act but a habit."

ARISTOTLE

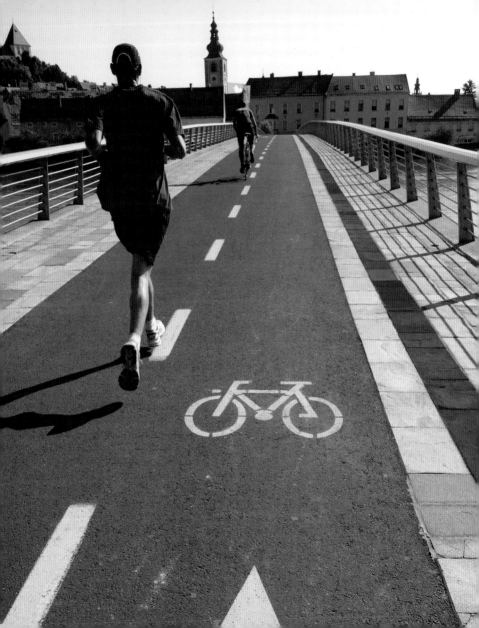

WEEK FOUR: YOUR TRAINING PROGRAMME AND DIARY

MON	7 mins brisk walk, 3 mins jog, repeat x3 (total 30 mins). Make sure you get warm on the brisk walk so you are ready for your run.
TUE	Rest.
WED	5 mins walk, 7 mins jog, 5 mins walk (total 17 mins). Stay focused on your jog and run at an easy and steady pace.
THU	Rest.
FRI	7 mins brisk walk, 3 mins jog, repeat x3 (total 30 mins).
SAT	Rest.
SUN	Rest or stretching.

THIS WEEK

 DO – Try to eat something nutritious (eg. a piece of fruit, porridge with cottage cheese, a handful of nuts or a toasted bagel with peanut butter) within 20 minutes of finishing exercise.

 CONSIDER – How many caffeine drinks you are having per day. Caffeine dehydrates your body.

 DON'T – Run in icy or snowy conditions as you could easily slip and injure yourself. It is possible to run on snow-covered grass fairly safely but this could be the time to use a treadmill.

REWARD

Have a cheat day. Eat and drink whatever you like and don't do any exercise.

sessions will simply become second nature to you. Just as you get up to clean your teeth and shower every morning without thinking about it, so you will soon be pulling on your shorts and heading out of the door for a jog without thinking about it.

Getting to that stage is easy enough. You should already be scheduling your training sessions into your day. Obviously there may be occasions when it's simply impossible to fit in a session so keep your training strategy flexible enough to be able to accommodate change for when life gets in the way. Don't beat yourself up if you have to miss a session but do not let this happen easily or the habit-forming process will be broken.

Find a time of the day that suits you best for training. You may prefer to run in the morning, "To get it out of the way", or you may like running later when the family is fed and settled in for the evening. Schedule in exercise according to your lifestyle and see what works best for you. For instance, if you normally run at night but you really enjoy winding down over a few drinks with colleagues on Friday after work, there's no need to compromise: swap your run to lunchtime and still enjoy your drinks. Running doesn't have to take over your life; it is something to add to it.

Varying your running routes is a good way to keep your enthusiasm levels up. The easiest thing to do,

66days

It takes an average of 66 days to form a habit. Although this is the average time it takes to turn something new into automatic behaviour a habit can form quicker for some or take considerably longer for others – so stick at it and exercise will soon become a habit for you. (6)

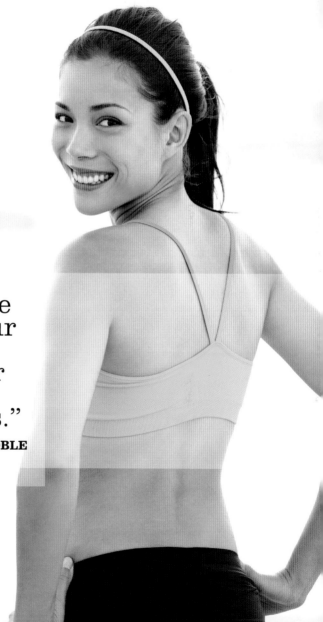

"First we
make our
habits
then our
habits
make us."

CHARLES C NOBLE

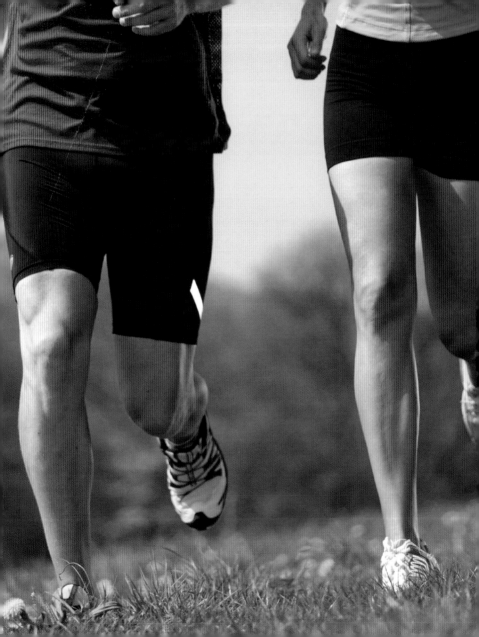

How many people get enough sleep?

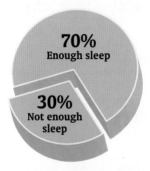

70%
Enough sleep

30%
Not enough sleep

Thirty per cent of working adults do not sleep enough (defined as less than six hours on average per day) according to a US survey.

A lack of sleep is associated with various health problems and makes it particularly difficult to train hard and get fit so make sure your lifestyle allows you to be part of the 70 per cent. (7)

especially when you start, is simply to head out of your front door and get moving. Walk/run half your session 'out', turn around and walk/run the other half of the session 'back'. So, for instance, on Friday's session this week (30 minutes in total) you turn at the 15-minute mark and head home. If it is not safe to run where you live (eg. because of heavy traffic), or you'd prefer different surroundings, then head somewhere peaceful such as nearby a park, lake, forest or to the coast. Try to run on flat routes as much as is possible (introduce hills gradually into your sessions when you feel ready). Tarred or paved areas are good for the stability they offer, although cut grass areas in parks offer a bit of relief from the jarring on your joints. Avoid fields with heavy grass and sand (eg. beaches) as both surfaces will slow you down and make it difficult for you to build up a steady running rhythm.

Another way to maintain the momentum is to find a training buddy. It's a lot harder to skip a session if you know your friend is waiting at the bottom of the road for you. And the amazing thing about training with someone else is that it's very rare you will both be feeling flat at the same time, so when you are down you'll be encouraged along and vice versa. If you think a training buddy is for you then find someone of about the same fitness level if possible. Whether it's a neighbour, a friend, sister or brother, you'll be surprised how many people there will be out there who'd like to help you in your challenge over the next few weeks.

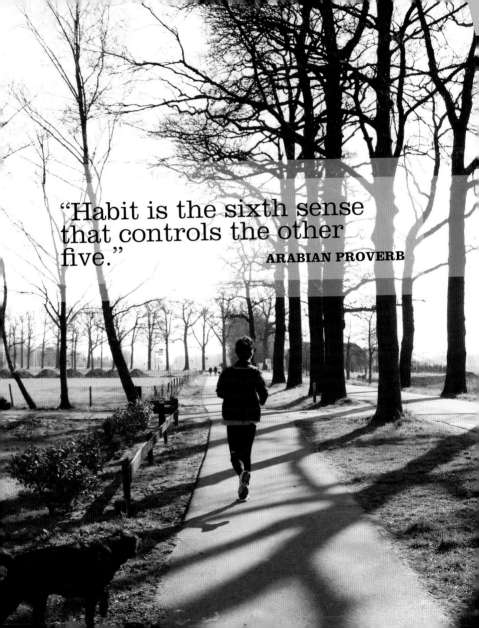

"Habit is the sixth sense that controls the other five."

ARABIAN PROVERB

that's it!

Week four completed

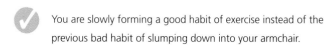 You are slowly forming a good habit of exercise instead of the previous bad habit of slumping down into your armchair.

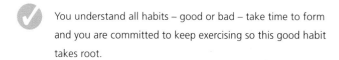 You understand all habits – good or bad – take time to form and you are committed to keep exercising so this good habit takes root.

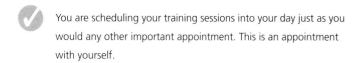 You are scheduling your training sessions into your day just as you would any other important appointment. This is an appointment with yourself.

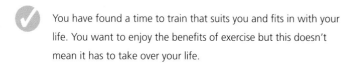 You have found a time to train that suits you and fits in with your life. You want to enjoy the benefits of exercise but this doesn't mean it has to take over your life.

Your notes at the end of the week

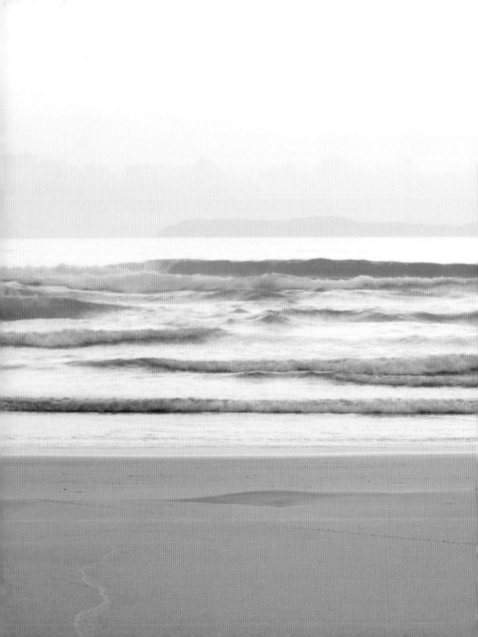

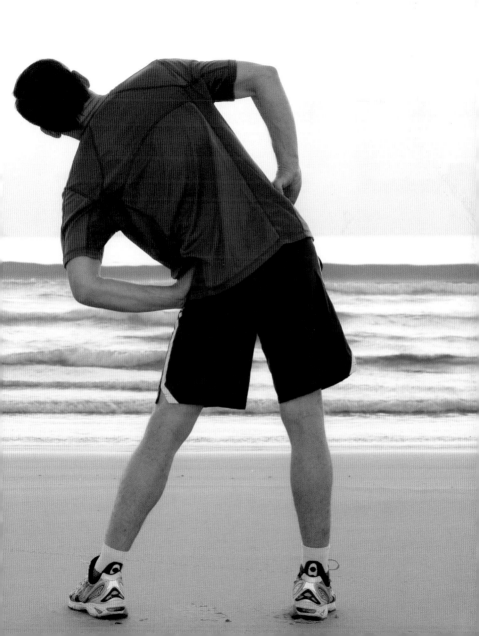

week five

Getting into the fitness groove

Running should be feeling easier and smoother. Enjoy the rhythm of it…

Although we are only a few weeks into the programme and there has only been a limited amount of running so far, you probably have started to feel some improvement to your rhythm already. Granted, you won't be leaping around like an Olympic gazelle just yet, but a bit of that original stiffness and awkwardness – your running rustiness – should have been shaken out of your legs and body.

The best way to improve at anything is to actually do it and so it is with running. Simply put, the best way to get better at running is to get out and actually run. However, there are still a few small things you can look at to help with the efficiency of your running style.

There is absolutely no need to get all technical and start adjusting this little thing and that little thing as if you are a professional golfer in search of the perfect swing. The main thing is to simply remain relaxed when you are running. It's easy, especially when you are just starting out or struggling during a run, to tense

YOUR AIM THIS WEEK

Is to ensure that you remain loose and relaxed when you are running.

It is not necessary to get caught up in the technical and scientific details of technique at this stage. Concentrate on keeping relaxed – particularly your neck and shoulders – and avoid tensing up your body as you run.

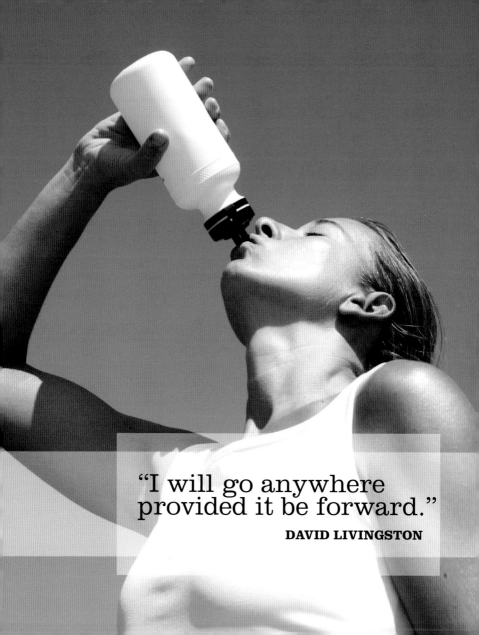

"I will go anywhere provided it be forward."

DAVID LIVINGSTON

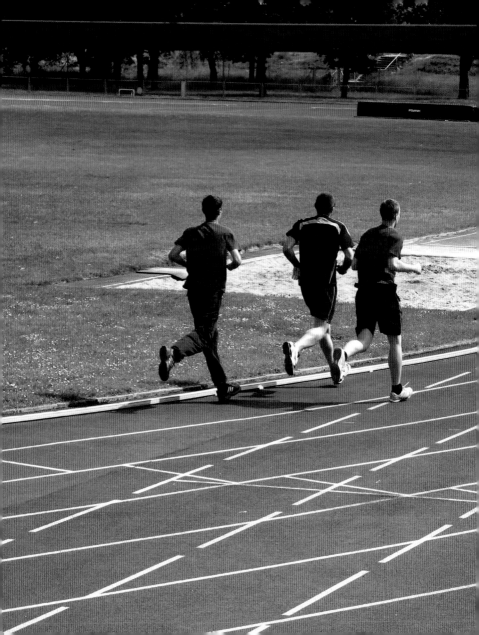

WEEK FIVE: YOUR TRAINING PROGRAMME AND DIARY

		YOUR DAILY NOTES
MON	6 mins brisk walk, 4 mins jog, repeat x3 (total 30 mins).	
TUE	Rest. Days off are even better when you feel like you deserve them, eh?	
WED	5 mins walk, 9 mins jog, 5 mins walk (total 19 mins). There is still some walking but you are now starting to jog for a decent time.	
THU	Rest.	
FRI	6 mins brisk walk, 4 mins jog, repeat x3 (total 30 mins). You can up the pace slightly on your walks if you are feeling comfortable.	
SAT	Rest. Remember your rest days are important so don't be tempted to do extra sessions.	
SUN	Rest or stretching.	

THIS WEEK

 DO – Carry a small water bottle on the longer runs so you can rehydrate. There are belts that will hold a bottle if you'd prefer not to hold it as you run.

 CONSIDER – A couple of easy healthier meat options like choosing white meat for red meat, or eating fish twice a week.

 DON'T – Start comparing yourself to others. Focus on your own goals.

REWARD

Treat yourself to some new exercise kit.

up your muscles. There's also a subconscious feeling that by straining you are somehow putting more into your workout as if are you going to get to the end quicker. Nothing could be further from the truth.

Relax, keep trusting your body, and your run will be a lot more enjoyable and you will reduce the stiffness in your joints and muscles. You don't need to look like a rag doll flopping along the road but if you feel yourself tensing up, simply breathe out deeply a couple of times and you will feel the looseness coming back to your body. If necessary stop running altogether, shake out your limbs one by one and give your neck a gentle roll.

In particular be aware of keeping your upper body relaxed and your neck and shoulders loose, as tension here can easily transfer itself to the rest of your body. You'll probably first become aware of this happening if you feel your face straining (not a good look either!). If you do feel your face tightening up, then straighten up your body and bring a smile to your face – you'll be amazed how this looseness just as quickly spreads through your other limbs and your running becomes smoother.

If you haven't already done so, this is the time to buy some proper running shoes (and some smart kit if you're feeling keen). While it's not impossible to train for and run a 5 km race in normal sports shoes

30mins

When running at a pace of 8 kph (5 mph) for 30 minutes a person weighing 56 kg (125 pounds) will burn 240 calories, while for someone weighing 70 kg (155 pounds) it is 298 calories, and at 84 kg (185 pounds) it is 355 calories. Figures are the same for circuit training, while swimming breaststroke burns 300, 372 and 444 calories respectively. For cycling at 19-22 kph (12-14 mph) the calories burnt are 240, 298 and 355. (8)

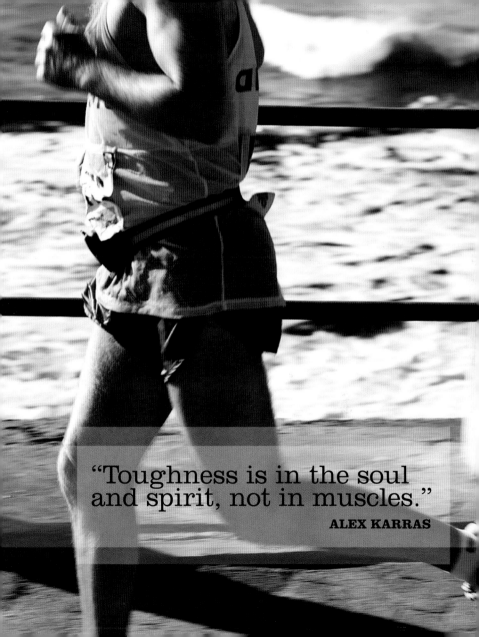

"Toughness is in the soul
and spirit, not in muscles."

ALEX KARRAS

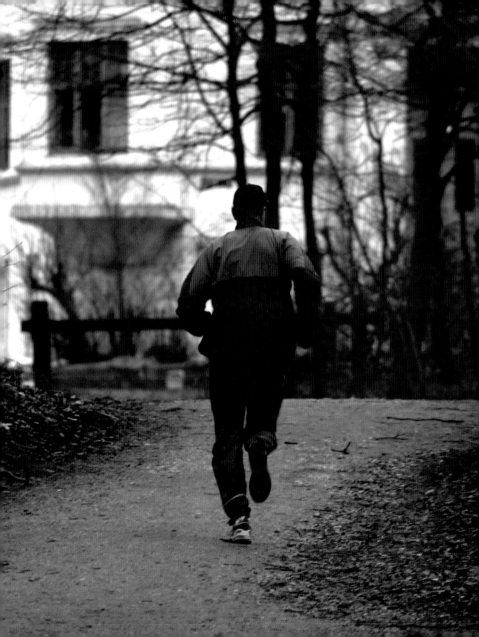

it certainly isn't advisable as they aren't built for running and therefore won't give you the support you need. As such you are much more likely to pick up an injury.

But which shoes to buy? Running shoes aren't cheap but you certainly don't have to spend a fortune to get a decent pair. Find a shop that specializes in running, or a sports store with a specialist running department and explain to one of the staff that you have just started running and need some advice. A good store will be able to check your running style and find a pair of shoes offering the right amount of support, cushioning and comfort. Many runners either pronate (ie. their foot rolls inwards when it lands) or over-pronate (ie. their foot rolls outwards). Staff will be able to test your running style and recommend a shoe that suits your needs.

As for kit, again it's certainly not impossible to run 5 km with any old pair of shorts or leggings and a baggy T-shirt. However, built-for-purpose running kit is designed using breathable material that operates better in different weather conditions. Wear underwear made of natural fibres that will breathe and reduce chaffing, or better still wear shorts with a built-in gusset. For women runners a sports bra is essential for comfort and support, and to minimize movement of the breasts. A good sports bra will also absorb sweat and not cut into your body as you run.

Calories in drinks

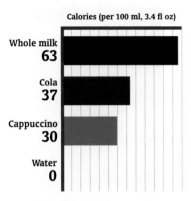

Calories (per 100 ml, 3.4 fl oz)

Whole milk **63**

Cola **37**

Cappuccino **30**

Water **0**

It's easy to rack up the calories you consume in drinks each day. Don't cut back and become dehydrated, just balance the type of drinks you enjoy. The chart shows figures for a glass of milk, Coca-Cola and a Starbucks cappuccino with whole milk. (9)

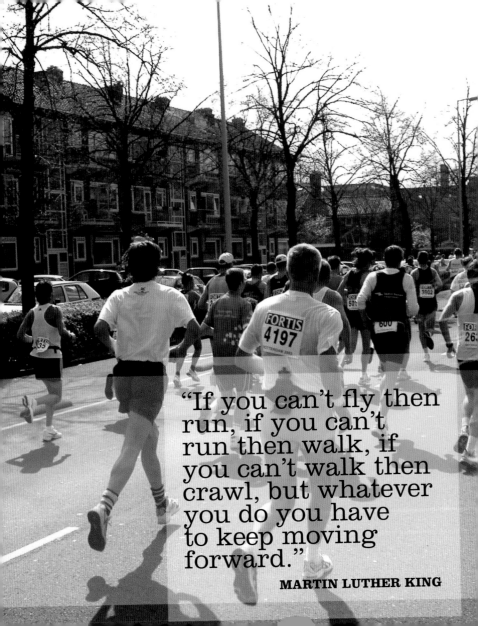

"If you can't fly then run, if you can't run then walk, if you can't walk then crawl, but whatever you do you have to keep moving forward."

MARTIN LUTHER KING

that's it!

Week five completed

 You are now in the training groove.

 You know the best way to get better at something is to do it, so keep on running and you will keep getting better.

 You know the best way to improve your technique is to stay loose and relaxed, in particular your neck and shoulders, so relax and trust your body to lead the way.

 You should have bought some proper running shoes and kit. The correct equipment will help you run better, feel better and it will help you avoid injuries.

Your notes at the
end of the week

week six

Start to enjoy the benefits

You'll already be starting to feel better and fitter. This is what you've been working for...

There's an example of a man who so loved takeaways and meeting his friends for a beer that he decided to take up exercise. "Hang on," you might be thinking, "that doesn't make the slightest bit of sense." Ah, but you see, his logic was blindingly simple, if a little odd: "As I get older all this fried food and beer is adding weight to my stomach I don't want, so it's either give up what I love or take up some exercise that allows me to continue eating and drinking what I please".

Now, while he realized this sort of argument was unlikely to be found in any fitness manual, he figured that doing something was better than doing nothing at all. He slowly started exercising and even began to enjoy it, and then one day in the office canteen he found himself ordering a healthy chicken rice and salad instead of the usual burger and fries. It wasn't as if he had suddenly become all pious and 'found health and fitness', it was simply that the running was having added positive effects and his body wanted something better to fuel this new-found exercise.

YOUR AIM THIS WEEK

Is to remain focused on your training and the end goal, and enjoy the benefits of exercising you may already be feeling.

Do not try to force changes in your life at this stage – just keep concentrating on the end goal and the other benefits will eventually come as a by-product of your good work.

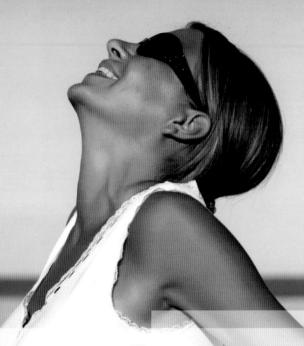

"By working hard
you get to play
hard, guilt-free."

JIM ROHN

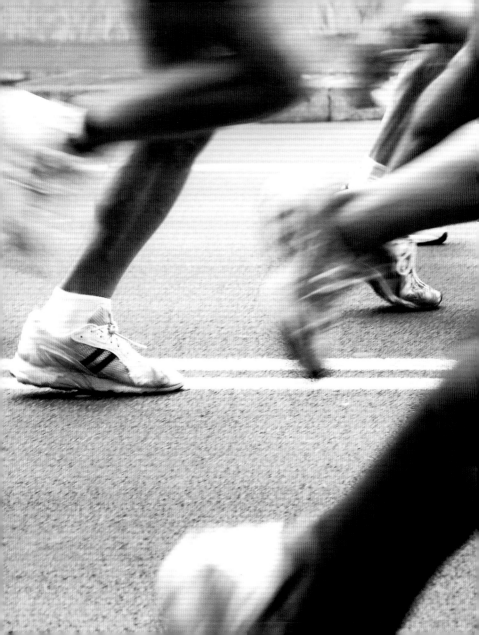

YOUR DAILY NOTES

MON	5 mins brisk walk, 5 mins jog, repeat x3 (total 30 mins).	
TUE	Rest.	
WED	5 mins walk, 11 mins jog, 5 mins walk (total 21 mins). Your long run is getting longer each week so stay focused.	
THU	Rest.	
FRI	5 mins brisk walk, 5 mins jog, repeat x3 (total 30 mins).	
SAT	Rest. Enjoy another couple of rest days after another good week of exercising.	
SUN	Rest or stretching.	

THIS WEEK

 DO – Keep your body tall over your hips, and avoid leaning forward or hunching your shoulders as your run. Look forward not down, keep your hands relaxed, and maintain a smooth stride.

 CONSIDER – Eating a nutritious breakfast (eg. porridge or fruit with yoghurt) every day. You've heard it before but it's certainly the most important meal of the day.

 DON'T – Allow yourself to become dehydrated when exercising. As you start to spend more time exercising you will need to start sipping water during your breaks.

REWARD

Book an Indian head massage.

Setting a goal (such as running 5 km) will set your subconscious to attract things to support the goal. As you get into training and maintaining focus on the goal, you may find yourself drawn to new strategies relating to nutrition, kit, or running techniques and so on.

As we stressed at the start, trying to change too much in your life at the same time is simply likely to lead to you giving up altogether. Starting exercise is a positive step already so there's no need to change everything. However, as the story above highlights, other positives are likely to follow. You may have already found yourself skipping your 'one for the road' glass of wine because you want to feel clear headed for your run in the morning, or maybe you have started drinking more water in the day. Don't force changes, no matter how enthusiastic you may be feeling, simply keep focused on training and the end goal and these other positives will start to follow.

For now, enjoy the benefits you are hopefully starting to feel already from exercising, such as sleeping better, waking up feeling more refreshed (if a little stiff) and feeling less jaded during the working day.

Now onto your target goal: you running 5 km. There are still a few weeks to go, plenty of time to get those muscles ready, so if you haven't already done it then now is the time to start thinking about where you will complete your challenge.

5days

Now you have started exercising you are well on your way to meeting guidelines set out by many government health experts — adults aged over 18 should exercise at moderate intensity for 30 minutes at least five days per week. The exercise does not need to be consecutive but should be in bouts of at least 10 minutes at a time. (10)

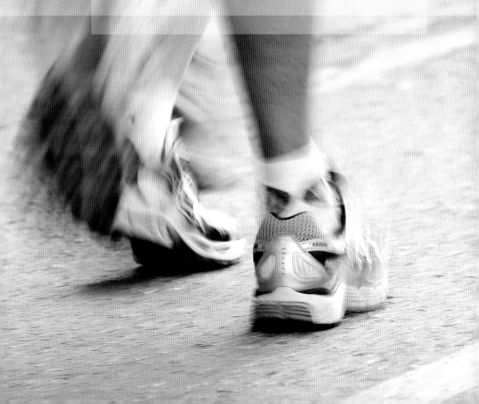

"It is remarkable how ones wits are sharpened by physical exercise."

PLINY THE YOUNGER

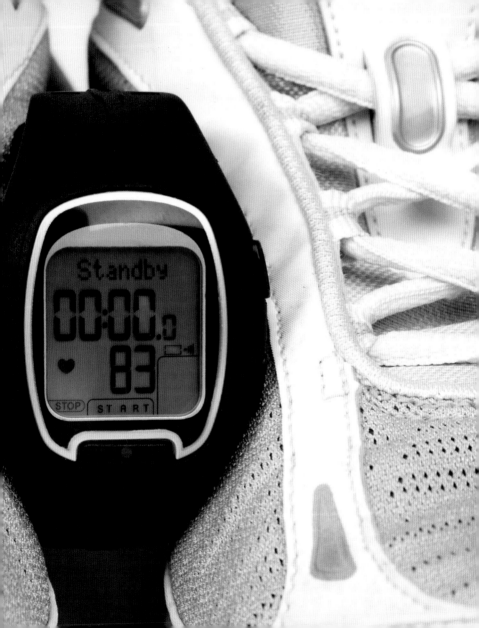

Calories burnt in 30 mins

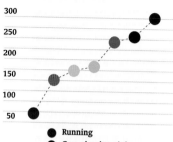

●	Running
●	Gym circuit training
●	Swimming
○	Cycling
◐	Mowing the lawn
◉	Walking
●	Ironing

Different activities use up varying amounts of energy and it's worth noting that even some daily activities help keep you healthy.

The chart shows figures for a walking lawn mower, brisk walking at 6.5 kph (4 mph), moderate cycling at 19-22 kph (12-14 mph), swimming at a pace of 46 metres (50 yards) a minute, and running at 9.5 kph (6 mph). (11)

The obvious thing, and certainly the most fun, is to identify an organized race that coincides with your target date and enter it. There are numerous organized races, all widely advertised, so there's likely to be one near you, although it would be more fun to celebrate your challenge with a weekend away somewhere that has a race. Grab your partner, family or friends (or all of them!) and head for the coast, mountains, big city, wherever it is that excites you the most. This will also give you an added spur in the coming weeks.

Entering an organized race gives you the added benefit of support, with water stations, marshals for road safety and, of course, the distance has been measured out exactly. Although there are some specific 5 km events, many of these races are likely be attached to a full or half-marathon race or linked to festival or special regional weekends where there are a series of different events. These races are usually well supported and are packed with people running their first race. Most races are held on weekends so there should be no problem finding one that falls on a Saturday or Sunday of Week 12 of your training programme.

If, however, you really do draw a blank with a race date, or just prefer to keep this as a solo exercise, there is no problem in organizing your own 'race'. It's easy enough to measure out your own 5 km in a car or on a bike in advance, then come 'race day' it's down to you, your legs and a stopwatch.

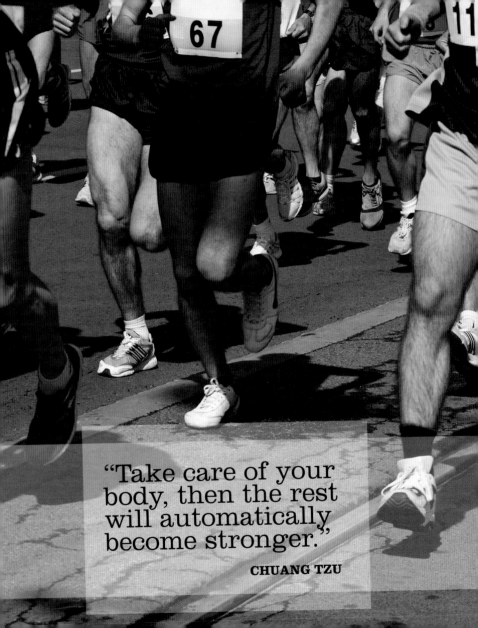

"Take care of your body, then the rest will automatically become stronger."

CHUANG TZU

that's it!

Week six completed

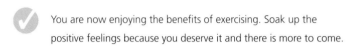 You are now enjoying the benefits of exercising. Soak up the positive feelings because you deserve it and there is more to come.

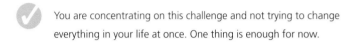 You are concentrating on this challenge and not trying to change everything in your life at once. One thing is enough for now.

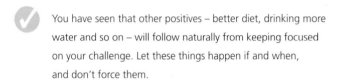 You have seen that other positives – better diet, drinking more water and so on – will follow naturally from keeping focused on your challenge. Let these things happen if and when, and don't force them.

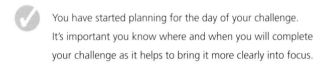 You have started planning for the day of your challenge. It's important you know where and when you will complete your challenge as it helps to bring it more clearly into focus.

Your notes at the
end of the week

week seven

You're halfway there

Time to take stock. Think how far you've come in a short time…

You are now halfway towards your final target of a 5 km race. It's possible you are feeling a bit apprehensive that you are not making progress fast enough and are worried you won't be able to make it. A run of 5 km when you only ditched the pizza box a few weeks ago can still feel like a long way off.

If this is you then relax, trust in the programme and don't lose your enthusiasm. What you have done so far is set a solid base, simply shaking off the cobwebs as you start to get active again and start to build up the habit of exercise. You now have the ideal launch pad to push on towards the end goal.

Think back to where you were just a few weeks ago when even closing your eyes and committing to this 12-week challenge felt like a big step. Remember how far you have come – and it really hasn't taken that long has it? Even in this short time you have probably already started to feel better both physically and mentally. Exercise improves the strength and fitness of

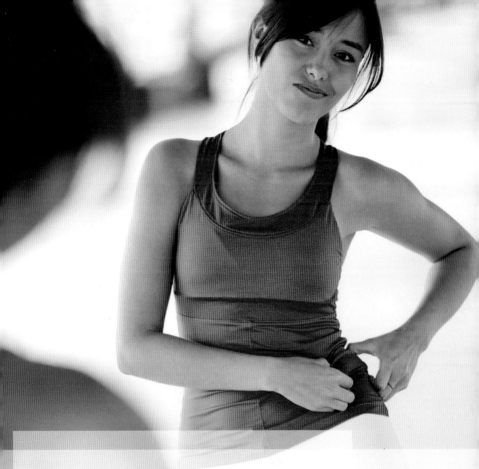

"Those who believe they can do something and those who believe they can't are both right."

HENRY FORD

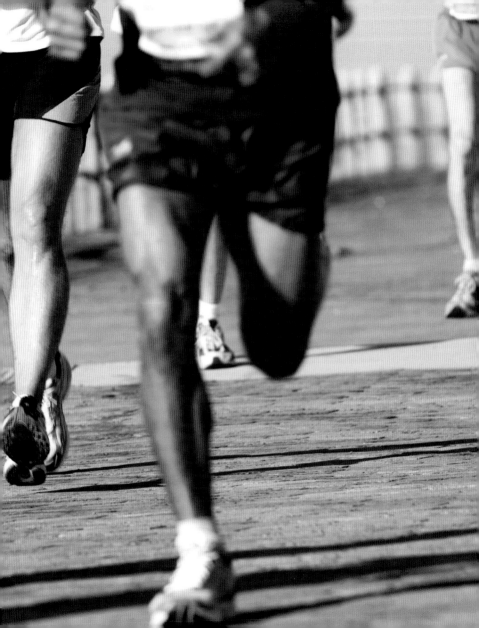

WEEK SEVEN: YOUR TRAINING PROGRAMME AND DIARY

		YOUR DAILY NOTES
MON	4 mins brisk walk, 6 mins jog, repeat x3 (total 30 mins). The first walk is getting shorter so stretch well before starting.	
TUE	Rest. Avoid the temptation to do extra sessions on your rest day. Let your body recover properly.	
WED	5 mins walk, 13 mins jog, 5 mins walk (total 23 mins). Use the first walk to stretch out your legs ready for your run.	
THU	Rest.	
FRI	4 mins brisk walk, 6 mins jog, repeat x3 (total 30 mins).	
SAT	Rest. Try to set aside a few minutes for a decent session of stretching today.	
SUN	Rest or stretching.	

THIS WEEK

 DO – Start to get more active in your everyday life such as walking up a couple of flights of stairs instead of taking the lift.

 CONSIDER – The amount of alcohol you drink the day before a session. There's nothing like a hangover to put you off exercising.

 DON'T – Start skipping sessions. This is a common problem a few weeks into a programme but consistent training is the only way to get results.

REWARD

Enjoy another cheat day – eat, drink and be merry.

your body, of course, but when done regularly it can also help to keep your mind alert and focused.

Be proud of your achievements so far. Worry less about tougher days and focus and repeat what you did on the good days. Keep a short-term memory for failures and a long-term memory for successes.

Read back over your notes for each session to remind yourself of what you have achieved already. We're sure a lot of them were similar to: "Struggled today, I'll never make it!" or "I couldn't even run for a few minutes before I had to stop for a breather." Compare them to what you are writing down for each session now and you should be able to measure your progress from these few comments.

Progress comes in small steps but all those small steps add up, so look back and congratulate yourself on what all those small steps have amounted to so far. Let's be honest, I'm sure a lot of people, maybe yourself included, never thought you'd even make it to the halfway stage. But now you're making steady progress.

If you are training with someone else try not to compare yourself all the time. A bit of healthy competition can help to spur you both on but don't let this simply become a contest; you didn't start this to be better than someone else, you started it for yourself. In particular, if your training buddy seems to

7, 8, 9

Most of us grow up being told that we need a 'good eight hours sleep' every night. Experts recommend seven to nine hours sleep a night for an adult – only you will know what is right for you. Try to get into a regular sleep pattern instead of trying to 'catch up' on the weekends as this re-sets your sleep cycle. (12)

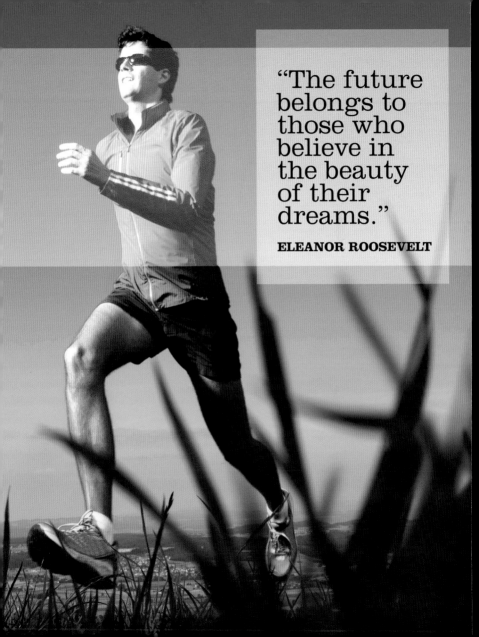

"The future belongs to those who believe in the beauty of their dreams."

ELEANOR ROOSEVELT

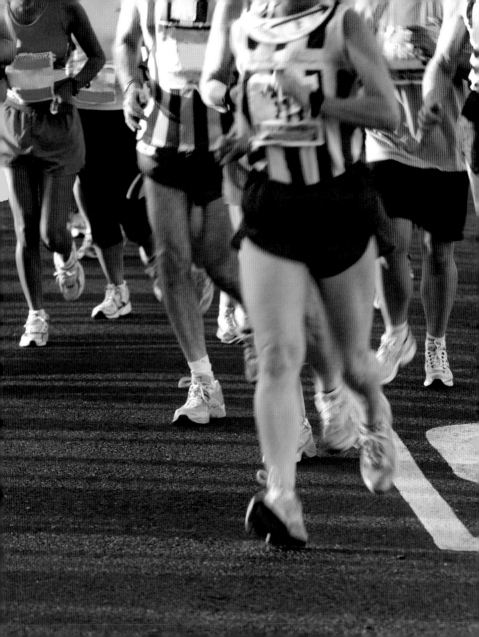

be making faster progress than you don't let it worry you. Everyone is different. The most important thing is that you are making progress.

Now you are at the halfway stage this is a good time to consider if you want to run to raise money for a charity. If you have entered one of the bigger events it's likely the event is actually organized to raise funds for a specific charity. Some of your entry fee may be earmarked for this charity although any extra you can raise will always be welcome, of course. Even if there is no specific charity aligned to your race you may still wish to use your efforts to raise some money. Most of us have a cause that is close to our heart for personal reasons and signing up with your chosen charity can also help give you an added incentive to complete what you have set out to do.

Charities will welcome your support, so simply contact your chosen one and explain what you are planning to do. Most charities are geared up for this and will have special packs with everything you'll need to help raise money such as sponsorship forms, posters, even security sealed collecting boxes if you want them. So what started out as a simple desire to get exercising again may now have snowballed into something a lot bigger. You've made steady progress with the programme, you're probably feeling fitter and healthier and, if you decide to sign up with a charity, you are raising money for a good cause as well.

Health benefits of fitness

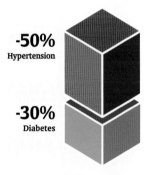

-50%
Hypertension

-30%
Diabetes

Exercising regularly reduces your risk of contracting many chronic diseases. These include Hypertension (50%), Ischaemic heart disease (40%), breast cancer (27%), a stroke (27%). (13)

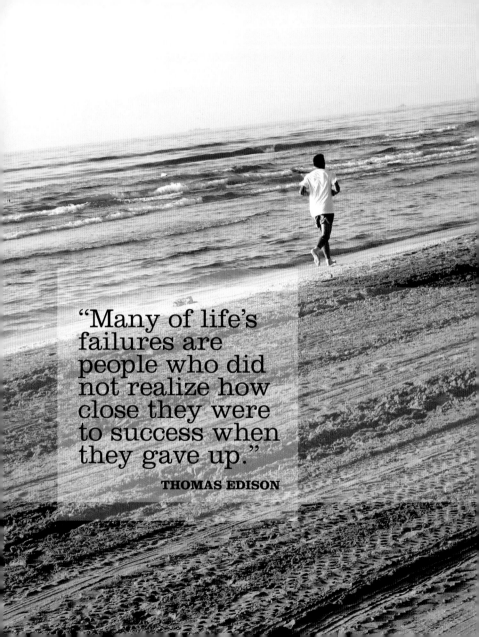

"Many of life's failures are people who did not realize how close they were to success when they gave up."

THOMAS EDISON

that's it!

Week seven completed

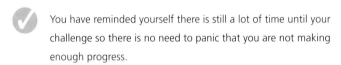 You have reminded yourself there is still a lot of time until your challenge so there is no need to panic that you are not making enough progress.

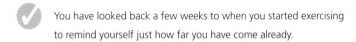 You have looked back a few weeks to when you started exercising to remind yourself just how far you have come already.

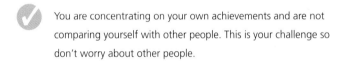 You are concentrating on your own achievements and are not comparing yourself with other people. This is your challenge so don't worry about other people.

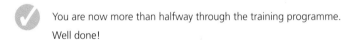 You are now more than halfway through the training programme. Well done!

Your notes at the end of the week

8 week eight

Recommit and look forward

Remind yourself why you started running and look ahead to the finish…

You are now entering the home straight of this 12-week programme. Now is the time to recommit to your goal of 5 km. Although the chances of giving up and returning to your armchair are lower now than they would have been in the earlier stages of the programme (after coming so far why give up now?) some people may still fall by the wayside so it's a good exercise to repeat.

Remember the day at the beginning when you told those people you had a target goal? Now is the time to do it again. Chances are that people are following your progress and asking about how you are getting on anyway so it'll be easy to slip into conversation, "Yes, just a few weeks to go until that race." As before, don't become the office bore, a simple mention in passing will do, if nothing else just so you hear it out loud again. Maybe this is the time to pin up a sponsorship form on the office notice board or e-mail friends and neighbours if you have chosen to run for a charity.

YOUR AIM THIS WEEK

Is to picture yourself successfully completing your challenge.

Your mind and body work together so this week is all about filling in the details of your success. 'See' yourself at the start ready then imagine how strong you are as you tackle your challenge. Then 'feel' how good it is to have succeeded.

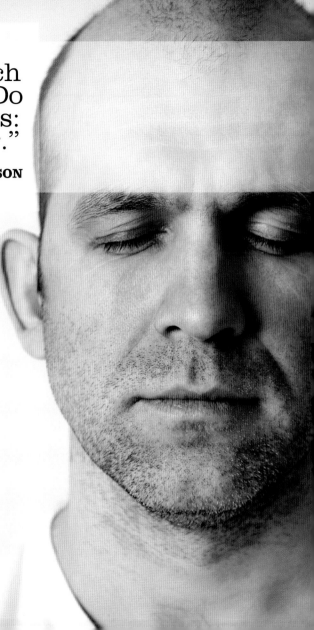

"Don't watch the clock. Do what it does: keep going."

SAM LEVENSON

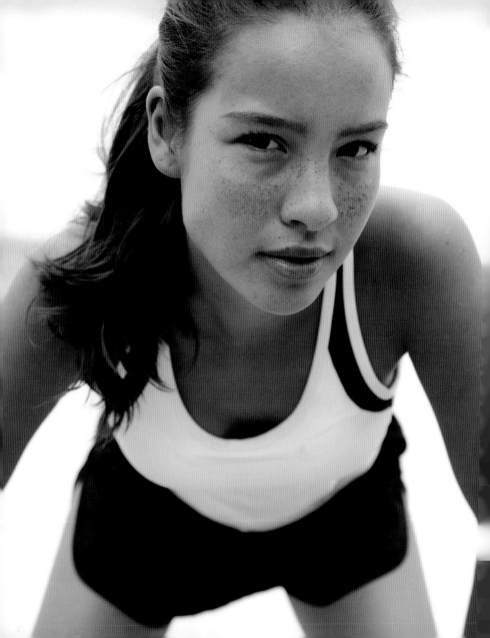

WEEK EIGHT: YOUR TRAINING PROGRAMME AND DIARY

MON	3 mins brisk walk, 7 mins jog, repeat x3 (total 30 mins). Remember to start slowly and keep your pace nice and steady.
TUE	Rest.
WED	5 mins walk 15 mins jog, 5 mins walk (total 25 mins). Use the walks to warm up and cool down.
THU	Rest.
FRI	3 mins brisk walk, 7 mins jog, repeat x3 (total 30 mins). The walks are now becoming important breaks to give you a breather.
SAT	Rest.
SUN	Rest or stretching. The next few weeks are crucial so make sure you use today to look ahead and make time for your future sessions.

THIS WEEK

 DO – Think about the intensity you are working at. Although you are probably fitter now, don't be tempted to push yourself harder. It's not the end yet.

 CONSIDER – Increasing the amount of vegetables you eat. It's easy enough to add an extra spoonful or two of veg to your plate.

 DON'T – Start over-eating sugary food. As you exercise more your appetite will grow and it's easy to snack on chocolate and other sweet foods.

REWARD

Enjoy a big night out with friends and eat and drink what you like.

This is also a good opportunity to picture the end result again. Remember the visualization exercise at the beginning? Now is the time to repeat the exercise, except this time with a few more details added in. It is well known that the body and mind are interlinked in their workings. Your mind is constantly telling your body what to do; in fact every time you make a movement of any sort the instruction has to come from your mind. So let's get them working together!

As mentioned at the beginning of the book, you don't have to become a mind-over-matter master but thoughts in your head *will* influence you so it makes sense to concentrate on the positive not the negative. This sort of thing does not have to be technical or complicated. In fact you do this all the time without even thinking. If you are planning to get a new kitchen your mind will have been turning over the options for weeks before you actually buy one. You've probably gone through it in immense detail: pictured the colour of the tops, 'seen' the shape of the taps, 'smelt' the richness of the wood, 'felt' the smoothness of the metal handles. Your mind comes up with the end result and your body (and wallet) heads off to make it a reality.

You have already done the most important thing, which is to set a goal. Once a goal has been set and you keep focused then your mind and body will work together to get there (which is why we keep repeating 'keep your mind on the end result').

Sports drinks contain two important ingredients – electrolytes (they help your muscles and heart function) and carbohydrates. You can lose electrolytes through very long workouts and the carbohydrates may help provide extra energy. Try sports drinks to see if they are for you, although water will always be important for most active people. (14)

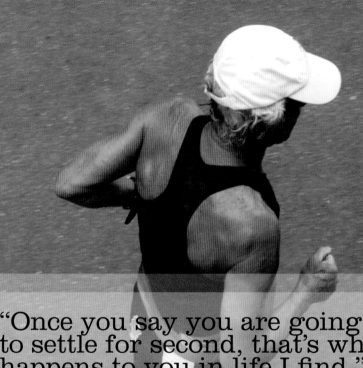

"Once you say you are going to settle for second, that's what happens to you in life I find."

JF KENNEDY

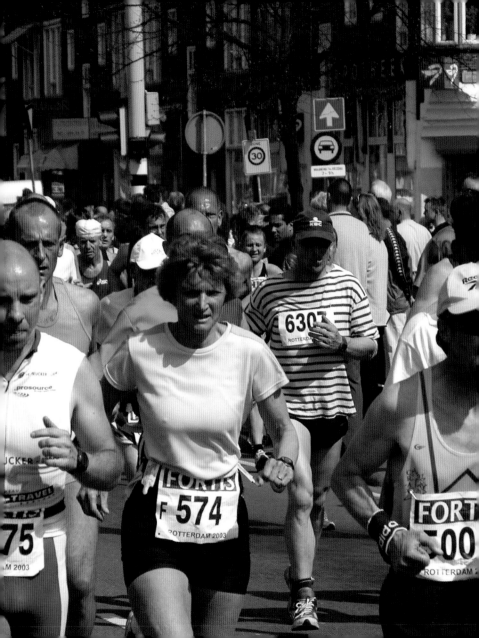

Calories in alcohol

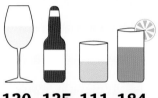

130
Glass of white wine

135
Bottle of beer

111
Gin with mixer

184
Alcopop

On a big night out it's easy to clock up the calories. The graphic shows figures for a 330 ml (11 fl oz) bottle of Stella Artois (4.8% abv), 175 ml (6 fl oz) glass of Jacob's Creek Chardonnay (13% abv), 25 ml (0.8 fl oz) of Bombay Sapphire (40% abv) and mixer, 275 ml (9 fl oz) WKD alcopop. (15)

Now let your mind paint a picture of a successful and enjoyable race day – and as you would with your new kitchen fill in the details. 'See' your friends and family at the start cheering you off, 'smell' the freshness in the air and 'sense' the anticipation of other runners at the start. Now picture yourself running along smoothly, maybe chatting to your running buddy or another friendly fellow runner. Feel the metres tick by with you feeling totally comfortable during the race and all the spectators cheering you on and clapping. Even that hill which you weren't too keen on is no problem as you climb it happily and reach the top.

Then 'see' the final stretch of the race; you are nearly there. If you used the reward element as part of your visualization you will 'remember' the reward (a beer, perhaps?) when it comes to reward time. This is known as a 'future memory', something you have 'remembered' but which hasn't happened yet! 'See' yourself crossing the line, relieved and happy, then join friends for a well-deserved pat on the back.

A lot of people, especially when they are starting out, dismiss this sort of thing but it takes just a few minutes at most and is as important as the physical work you have been doing. Visualization techniques are used by many top sportspeople because they are so powerful. The more you can 'see' and 'feel' your event, the more 'experienced' you will feel come race day. The conscious mind can blur real and imagined events.

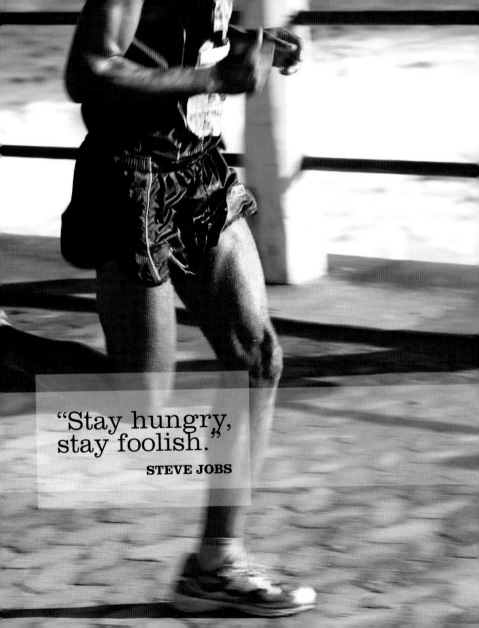

"Stay hungry,
stay foolish."
STEVE JOBS

that's it!

Week eight completed

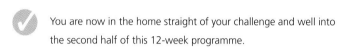

You are now in the home straight of your challenge and well into the second half of this 12-week programme.

You have recommitted yourself to your challenge by telling your friends, family and colleagues about your progress or maybe you have started to collect sponsorship if you have chosen a charity.

You recognize that setting the goal at the start was the most important thing you could have done and your mind and body will work together towards achieving that goal.

You have let your mind paint a full picture of your run on race day, filling in details to make the picture as complete as possible.

Your notes at the
end of the week

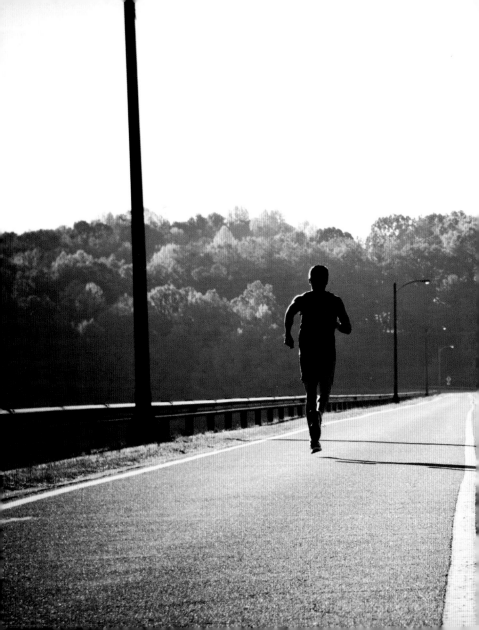

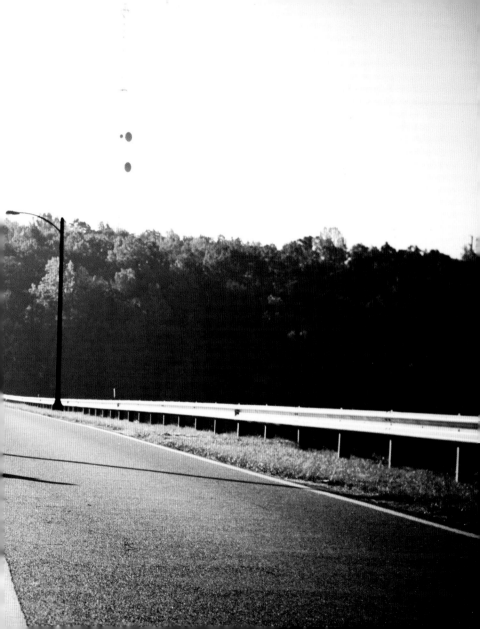

*9*week nine

Now push on towards your end goal

It's time to crank up the energy levels…

Earlier on in the programme we mentioned the importance of keeping yourself relaxed when you are running and trusting your body to find a style that suits it best. You have enough to concentrate on with simply getting fit enough for the end goal, so at this stage this is the best way for you to settle into running smoothly. But there are still a few easy tricks you can adopt and a few things you can take on board to help make your running easier and more enjoyable. As we said earlier, who would turn down the chance to get better results for less effort?

Unless you are from another planet you probably don't like running up hills. Or even seeing them ahead of you. No one does. There you are, running along happily and enjoying yourself and you turn the corner to see a long climb ahead of you. It's enough to make a grown man groan. It's a natural tendency but the worse thing you can do at this stage is tense up, so remember all the pointers from earlier about keeping your neck, shoulders and face relaxed. If you do tighten up then the tension will spread and your

YOUR AIM THIS WEEK

Is to look closer at your technique to see how this can help your running.

There is no need to become a technical guru overnight but spending a few minutes looking at ways that can fine-tune how you run can help you to run better with less effort. Anyone against that idea?

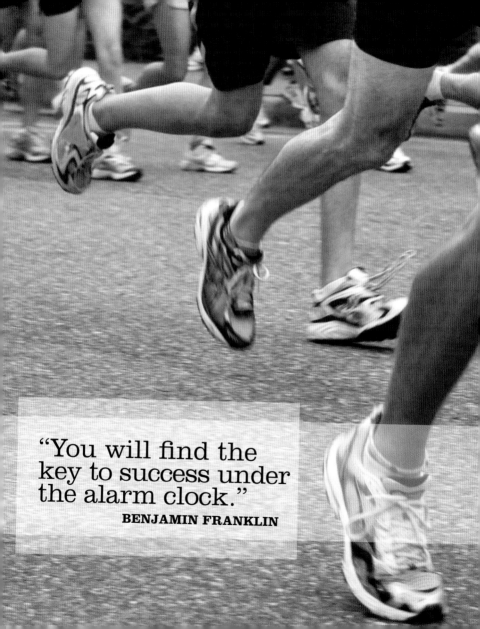

"You will find the
key to success under
the alarm clock."

BENJAMIN FRANKLIN

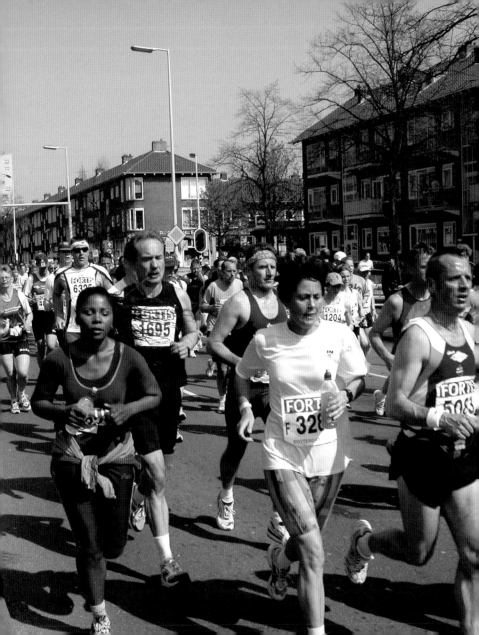

		YOUR DAILY NOTES
MON	2 mins brisk walk, 8 mins jog, repeat x3 (total 30 mins). Ensure you are stretched out before you start because the first walk is very short.	
TUE	Rest.	
WED	5 mins walk, 3 km jog, 5 mins cool down (total 10 mins and 3 km). Don't worry about your time as this is all about covering the distance.	
THU	Rest.	
FRI	Cross-train (eg. swimming or cycling). Do something different to avoid the boredom and to work different muscles.	
SAT	Rest.	
SUN	Rest or stretching.	

THIS WEEK

 DO – Re-evaluate the way you are running. Concentrate on keeping your style smooth and relaxed.

 CONSIDER – Introducing a bit more fruit into what you eat. Things like apples and bananas are ideal for busy people who always find they are eating on the go.

 DON'T – Use the rain as an excuse to skip a session. Running in the rain can actually be exhilarating as long as you keep warm.

REWARD

Block out an hour to yourself, then put your feet up and relax.

whole body will become rigid, making the hill climb even harder.

When you reach the hill don't crouch over as if you are in fear of the slope but keep your body upright and your eyes looking forward as this will help you stay loose. Some people do prefer to look down as they find that it helps them mentally because they can't see the hill (but always take care when looking down!). If you can somehow do this without tightening up then give it a go but the upright approach is preferable as being relaxed is the key.

You have probably found yourself taking shorter strides when you climb a hill, which is good as common mistakes when running uphill are to stretch out your strides further than usual and to lean forward. This is your subconscious effort to 'beat the hill' or at least 'get it over with as quickly as possible'. Again, these are perfectly natural tendencies but not good ones. Avoid this and accept you are inevitably going to slow down a bit when you are running uphill. It is like when you are driving a car; you often have to drop down a gear on a steep slope.

When going uphill try to maintain the same level of effort as you would when you are running on the flat and just accept it's natural to slow down. When you do get to the top don't be tempted to stop or slow down in relief at having made it, but keep going

4or9

Sugars and starches (carbohydrates) found in foods such as pasta, bread, cereal, fruit and vegetables have four calories per gram (0.14 oz) while fat is more than double at nine calories per gram (0.32 oz). Worth knowing when you're trying to get fit and healthy don't you reckon? (16)

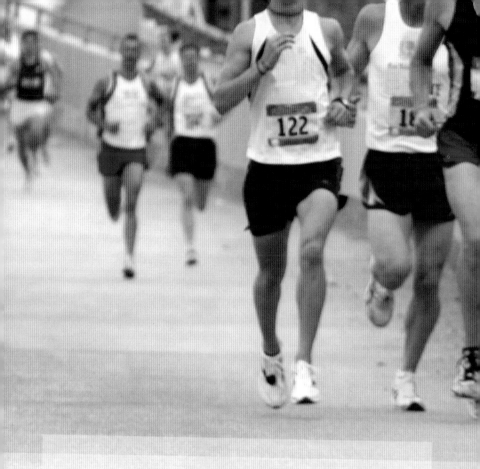

"Be miserable. Or motivate yourself. Whatever has to be done, it's always up to you."

WAYNE DYER

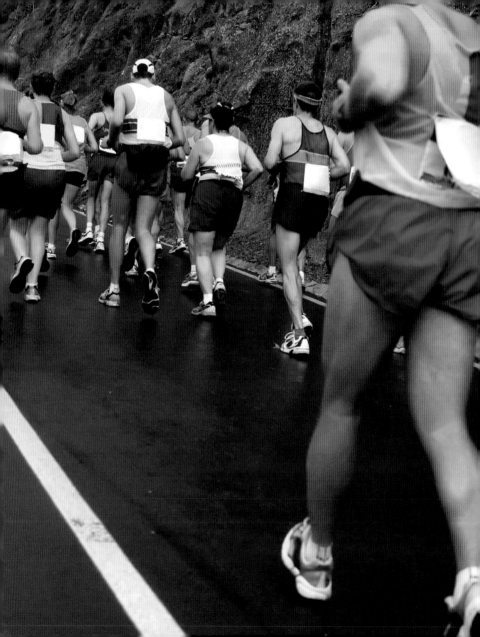

at the same effort level and you will quickly regain your breath. Finally, if you do find yourself walking up part of the hill or all of it, even at this stage in the programme, then that's fine as you will continue to improve over the coming weeks.

Ah, then there are the lovely downhill runs. Just as that feeling of dread sweeps over us when we see a hill climb ahead so we all love to see a nice stretch of downhill. A good way to get a few easy metres out the way, perhaps? But don't go charging down the hill like an excited bull. Instead, enjoy the ride and keep it as graceful as possible. Your body will naturally pick up a bit of pace because of gravity so go with it but don't force it.

Just as you should avoid the temptation to lean forwards when running uphill so you should avoid leaning backwards when running on a downward slope. Stay as upright as possible and try not to shuffle your feet. On the steeper downhills you may start to feel out of control as if your body is running away from you. When this happens ease up until you have built up more confidence. This is particularly relevant if you are running on a rough surface. Even a road, let alone a dirt or gravel track, may have a pothole or a loose stone you can slip on – not pleasant when you are careering downhill. Keep your eyes alert for such obstacles, and in a race, of course, for other runners.

A balanced diet

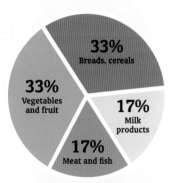

33%
Breads, cereals

33%
Vegetables and fruit

17%
Milk products

17%
Meat and fish

Try to maintain a balanced diet of the 'basic four food groups' in the proportions shown in the chart above and to eat from all of them every day. Also limit the amount of fats you include in your diet. (17)

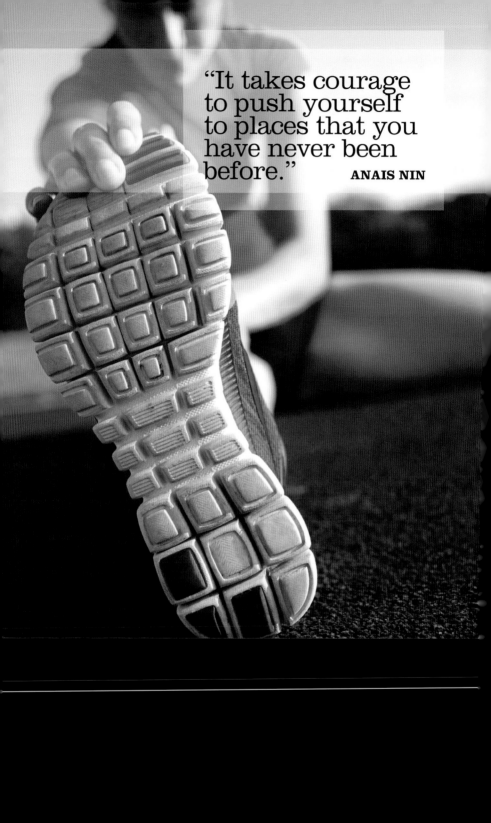

"It takes courage to push yourself to places that you have never been before." **ANAIS NIN**

that's it!

Week nine completed

 You have reminded yourself that the best thing to remember when training is to stay loose and relaxed.

 You know it is particularly important to keep relaxed and loose when running uphill. There is nothing to fear from a hill and over time you will dread those climbs less as they approach.

 You know it is important to take shorter strides and maintain an even level of effort when running uphill and accept you will slow down. Don't try 'to beat' the hills.

 You can learn to enjoy the extra pace that is naturally generated as you run downhill but you must not get carried away and start charging downhill like a wild bull.

Your notes at the
end of the week

10 week ten

Time to turn on the cruise control

**You're feeling fit and healthy. This running
is becoming a stroll in the park…**

By now running is probably becoming second nature
to you. Get up, pull on your shoes, shorts and T-shirt,
head out the door, run, stretch, home. Maybe you're
thinking: "Can't think why I didn't start this earlier
really? I'm feeling fitter and looking well, what can go
wrong?" Well, there are a couple of things that can
go wrong and as you are so close to your end goal
you need to guard against them carefully.

The first is worrying that you haven't done enough.
This can lead to a last-minute panic of thinking you
need to cram in some extra sessions on rest days or
do a 'bit extra' on the sessions planned. While this is
understandable, especially as you are so determined
to complete the 12-weeks successfully, it will actually
do more harm that good. The programme has been
designed to get you gradually to your goal (remember
the building blocks?) so if you have followed it
correctly then you will be fit and strong enough to
complete the run successfully when the day comes.
Extra sessions now, especially tough ones, will drain

YOUR AIM THIS WEEK

Is to guard against over-
confidence or worrying that
you have not done enough.

Over-confidence can mean
you push yourself too hard
in training, while worrying
that you have under-trained
could lead to you trying
to force in extra sessions.
Avoid both and trust the
programme.

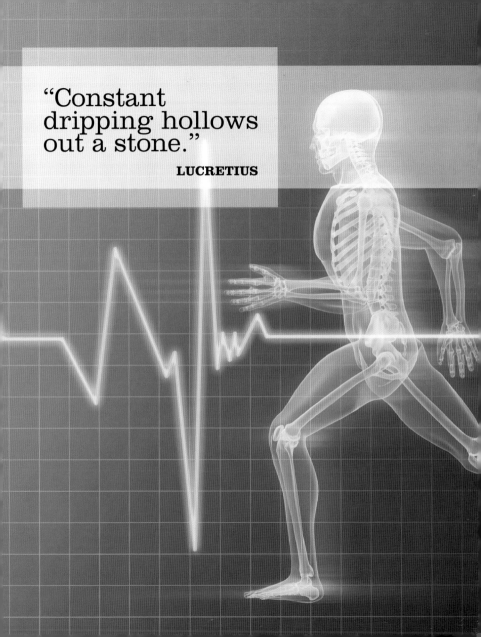

"Constant dripping hollows out a stone."

LUCRETIUS

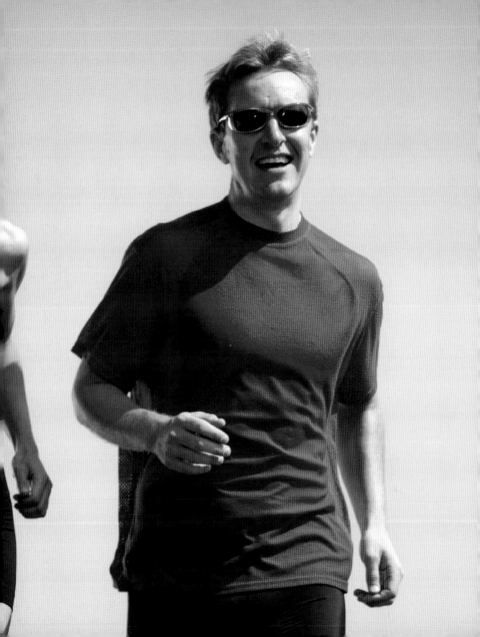

WEEK TEN: YOUR TRAINING PROGRAMME AND DIARY

		YOUR DAILY NOTES
MON	1 min brisk walk, 9 mins jog, repeat x3 (total 30 mins). Use the short walks to get used to drinking water during exercise.	
TUE	Rest.	
WED	5 mins walk, 20 mins jog, 5 mins brisk walk (total 30 mins).	
THU	Rest. A bit of stretching on your rest day is even more important now you are running so much.	
FRI	1 min brisk walk, 9 mins jog, repeat x3 (total 30 mins).	
SAT	Rest.	
SUN	Rest or stretching. Ensure you are warm before stretching out your muscles as you have a couple of important weeks ahead.	

THIS WEEK

 DO – Remind yourself why you started running and the success you have enjoyed already, if you 'can't be bothered' to train one day.

 CONSIDER – Running in the morning or when the sun sets during the summer months so you avoid the worst of the heat.

 DON'T – Start skipping your warm-ups and cool downs to save time when you exercise. These are important parts of the sessions.

REWARD

Block off a chunk of time one day – as much as possible – and do what you love the most.

your legs, could lead to injury and ruin all the hard work you have put in so far.

The same, incidentally, is true if you are feeling super strong. You may have progressed way more than you could have imagined but over-confidence can also lead to you doing too much at this stage instead of staying focused on the end result. There is an example of a man who trained really hard for a race. He stuck rigidly to the programme he had chosen because he trusted it would get him to his end goal, even to the extreme of driving the friends he trained with sometimes absolutely mad. But it worked. He shed loads of weight and started to get stronger and quicker. Then, two weeks before the race on a training run he declared to his friends that he was feeling strong and wasn't sticking to the planned pace that day. He charged off with his new-found confidence and finished the run way ahead of his training buddies. Two weeks later he failed to finish his target race because he was too drained from his training. Do you want to ruin weeks of hard work in the same way?

You may also be aiming for a particular time during your run. We have avoided discussion of this because the aim is to simply get you from the armchair to the end goal but it is inevitable that as you got stronger during the programme you may have set a specific time target. Nothing wrong with that, and good

17-19

Researchers in Australia and New Zealand found that people who drove after being awake for 17-19 hours performed worse than those who had a blood-alcohol level of 0.5 per cent — the legal limit for drivers in Australia and many European countries. It's not difficult to see that sleep is important for anyone who wants to focus on his/her health and fitness. (18)

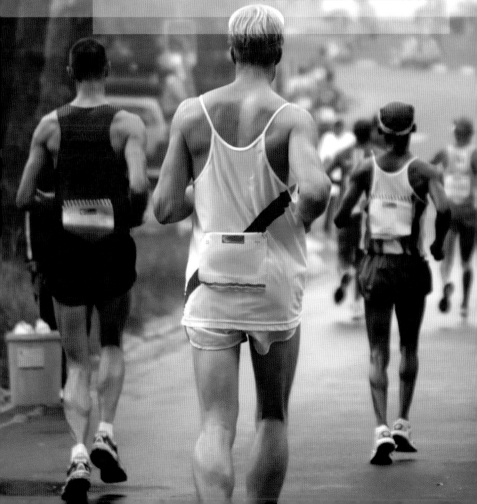

"Adopt the pace of nature:
her secret is patience."

RALPH WALDO EMERSON

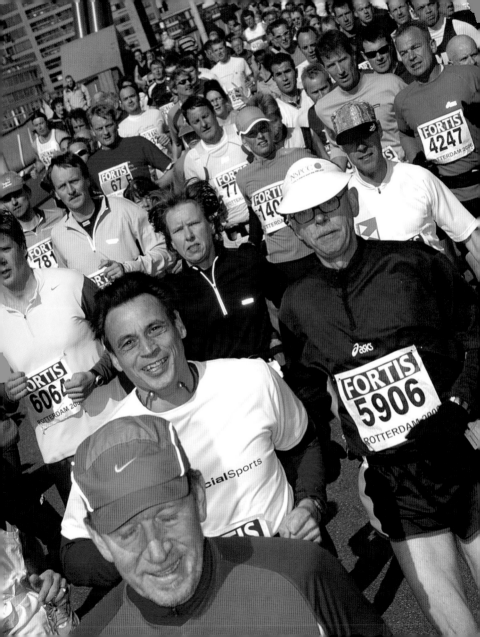

luck with it, but ensure first and foremost that you complete the race successfully. Rather keep focused on the end goal – the performance – and a desired outcome of a particular time should follow.

The human body

60%
Water

40%
Other

Around 55-60 per cent of your body is made up of water. Your brain is 70 per cent water, blood 83 per cent water and lungs nearly 90 per cent. Make sure you keep yourself topped up by drinking plenty of water throughout the day. (19)

One of the worst things that can happen at this stage is for you to pick up an injury or get sick. You already know stretching is one of the best things you can do to avoid injury, so continue to stretch before and after a training session and on your days off, too, if you can. In the event you do pick up an injury, though, it's important you rest as a couple of days off could give you time to recover. Do not train with an injury. If necessary get the injury checked out by a physio or a doctor. It is better for you to miss one or two sessions than to make the injury worse and fail to complete your end goal altogether.

Catching a common cold at this stage can be frustrating. The good news is that moderate regular exercise increases your immune system so your chance of picking up a bug is lower than it was before you started exercising. But Sod's Law and all that, eh? Be particularly strict about sticking to all the usual healthy things you do to avoid catching a cold (like washing your hands regularly etc). In addition, after a training session get in a bath or shower as soon as possible and put on warm clothing afterwards as your body temperature will drop quickly once you stop moving.

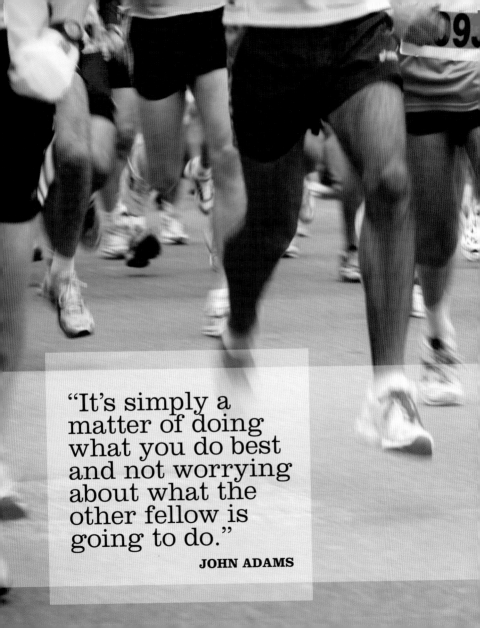

"It's simply a matter of doing what you do best and not worrying about what the other fellow is going to do."

JOHN ADAMS

that's it!

Week ten completed

 Running is starting to become second nature to you. Bet you can't believe you didn't start this earlier now.

 You have reminded yourself that if you have followed the programme then you will be in good shape for race day. There is no need to worry you have not done enough training and you need to do extra.

 You have also reminded yourself that even if you feel strong this is not the time to get carried away. Keep your eyes on the end goal and stick to the programme.

 You know that if you pick up an injury you must rest and if it persists seek a professional opinion from a doctor or a physio. Do not keep training with an injury.

Your notes at the end of the week

You're nearly there

It's time to start winding down and to concentrate on the race…

If you were a professional athlete then every day you could wake up, go training, eat and sleep, and repeat this routine over and over again without worrying about the other mundane stuff in life. Nothing would be left to chance and 100 per cent of your effort would be geared towards your end goal. Even some serious runners who aren't even professionals organize their lives around their most important races by doing things such as taking a few days off work, finishing early or even arranging help for important personal tasks so they can concentrate on being completely ready for their end goal.

Meanwhile back in the real world, where the rest of us live, there are children that need picking up from school, reports to be delivered on deadline to frantic bosses, and daily jobs to be done around the house. You can't control these responsibilities and then, just when you least want it, something else pops up like your car breaking down or your accountant rings and asks for all your tax receipts from five years ago.

YOUR AIM THIS WEEK

Is to realize that this is not the time to be taking on new projects even if you think they might help distract your nerves.

There are certain responsibilities we all have to continue to fulfil in our work, family and social life so keep those new projects on the back burner for a couple more weeks.

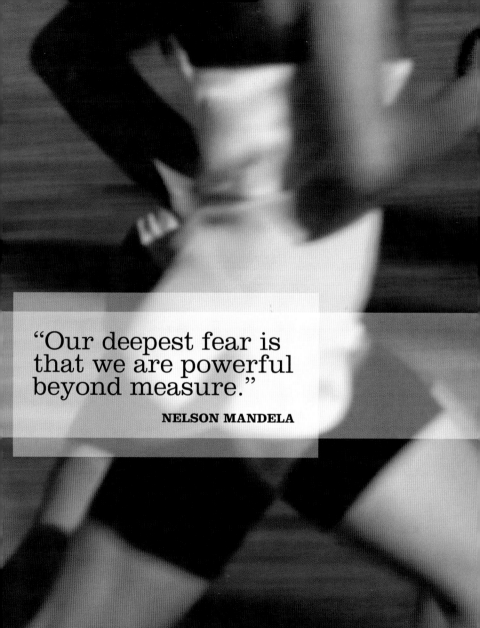

"Our deepest fear is that we are powerful beyond measure."

NELSON MANDELA

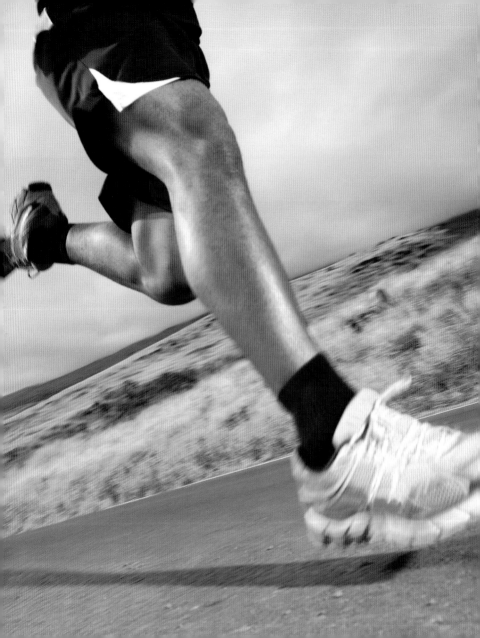

WEEK ELEVEN: YOUR TRAINING PROGRAMME AND DIARY

YOUR DAILY NOTES

MON	5 mins warm up, 5 mins slightly quicker jog, 5 mins walk (total 15 mins).
TUE	Rest.
WED	5 mins warm-up, 4 km jog, 5 mins cool down (total 10 mins and 4 km). Keep focused and relaxed during your run.
THU	Rest.
FRI	Cross-train (eg. swimming or cycling). Enjoy the change but don't push it too hard if it's something you are not used to doing.
SAT	Rest. Relax and avoid doing anything stressful because this is your last weekend before the big day.
SUN	Rest or stretching.

THIS WEEK

 DO – Start to look ahead to your race day and remind yourself that you are ready.

 CONSIDER – Going to a yoga class for some stretching on one of your rest days.

 DON'T – Panic and think you can improve things at this stage by pushing yourself extra hard in the next couple of weeks.

REWARD

Book a relaxing body massage.

This is the reality of life for most of us and it's probably the reason you couldn't fit exercise into your daily routine before. But now you have broken out of your pizza-armchair habit and are slowly getting fitter and healthier.

So although you can't control many of those things mentioned above you don't use them as excuses anymore and have still managed to get to the verge of your end goal: a 5 km race. But there are some things that you can control, so let's concentrate on those things.

This is certainly not the time to be taking on new projects. Yes, we're sure your garage needs cleaning out and the door to the shed needs fixing but they've both been like that for months so a couple more weeks won't really hurt, will it? And while the nice blue paint for the spare bedroom might be sitting in the shed (the one with the broken door) just waiting to go on the walls, don't be tempted to start that job until you have finished your 12-week programme either.

Doing jobs like these at a time like this is an easy thing to do because you are probably starting to become a little nervous about your challenge. After all, the run is only a few days away and you have worked so hard to get to this point so it is perfectly natural. And when we get nervous we take on tasks

36°C

Be particularly careful when exercising in hot weather. Once the temperature rises to 36°C (97°F) it is recommended you cancel your session or postpone it to a cooler part of the day as the heat will put a lot of stress on your body. [20]

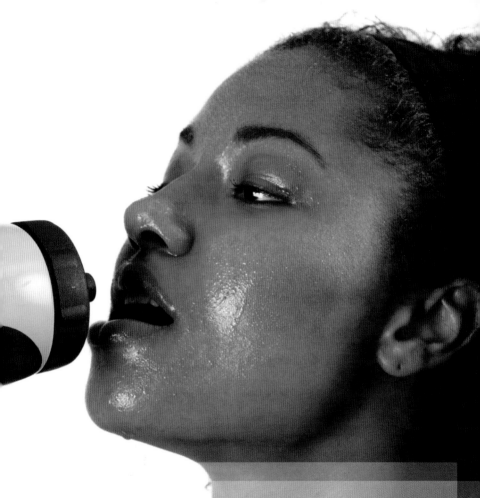

"For success, attitude is equally important as ability."

HARRY F BANKS

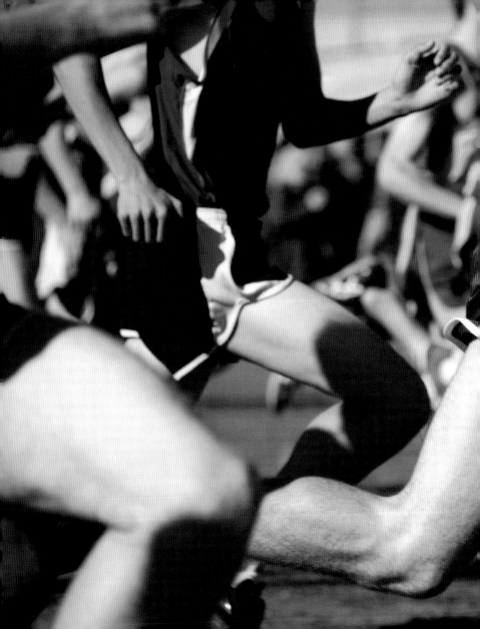

A balanced meal

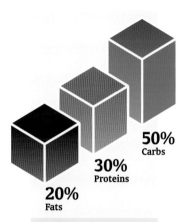

50%
Carbs

30%
Proteins

20%
Fats

Try to balance all food elements with every meal you eat in line with the figures shown in the chart above.

Carbohydrates include rice, bread, fruits and vegetables, proteins come from meat, fish, milk products and eggs, while nuts, avocados, green olives, fish oil and olive oil are a good source of fats. (21)

like these to distract our mind. But right now you need to keep what you are doing to the minimum and concentrate on the race ahead.

There is no need to worry, because if you have been following the programme correctly then you will be on track to complete your challenge so there really is nothing to worry about. This is just nervous excitement. You may not be able to get rid of all the butterflies in your stomach but you can get them to fly in unison with you. Just not while you are cleaning out the garage please.

So do the things that have to be done in your life and quietly ignore those things that can be put off until later (at least for a few more days until the race is over). If your partner starts moaning just tell them that relaxation is just as important as training when it comes to this programme. They probably won't agree, of course, but just smile and blame this book, we don't mind.

This is also the time to make sure you are getting enough sleep every night (you can record that late film to watch later), to be drinking lots of water and easing up on the alcohol. This doesn't mean you have to become a monk – a couple of beers won't hurt – but this isn't really the time to head out on the town and see if you can still drink like you could in your student days.

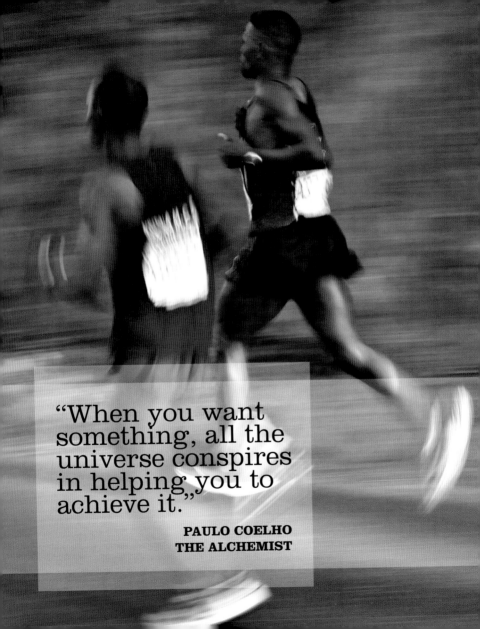

"When you want something, all the universe conspires in helping you to achieve it."

**PAULO COELHO
THE ALCHEMIST**

that's it!

Week eleven completed

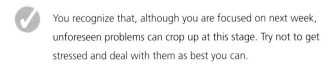 You recognize that, although you are focused on next week, unforeseen problems can crop up at this stage. Try not to get stressed and deal with them as best you can.

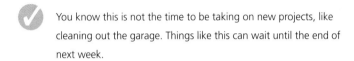 You know this is not the time to be taking on new projects, like cleaning out the garage. Things like this can wait until the end of next week.

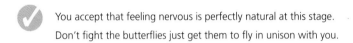 You accept that feeling nervous is perfectly natural at this stage. Don't fight the butterflies just get them to fly in unison with you.

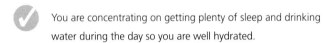 You are concentrating on getting plenty of sleep and drinking water during the day so you are well hydrated.

Your notes at the end of the week

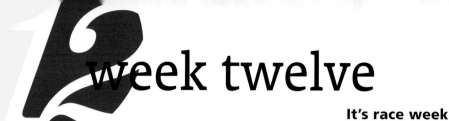

week twelve

It's race week

**This is what you've been aiming for.
You're ready for your race...**

This is it then. After weeks of hard work you are now on the verge of completing your 12-week challenge. As we have emphasized before, if you have followed the programme correctly you will be well prepared for your race and have nothing to worry about. So just relax and relish the moment.

There are only a couple of sessions this week so enjoy them, making sure to keep nice and loose. Depending on whether your chosen race is on Saturday or Sunday you will have two or three days of rest leading up to it. These rest days are important for your body and will ensure that you are fresh come your big day so treat them with respect. However, a little bit of gentle stretching is recommended on these days so your muscles don't tighten up.

Make sure you are prepared and get everything ready for the race well ahead of time. Go through the checklist below and get you bag ready early so there are no last-minute panics to distract you.

YOUR AIM THIS WEEK

Is to go out with a smile on your face and complete your challenge successfully.

This is what you have worked so hard for over the past 12 weeks. Now is the time to put all that training to good use and run your race – and to enjoy yourself as you do it.

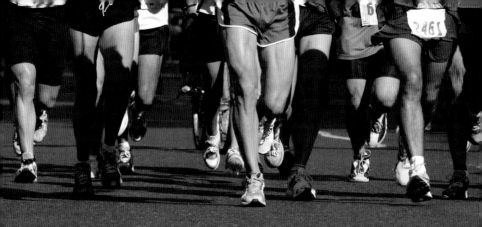

"The world you desire can be won. It exists... it is real... it is yours."

AYN RAND, ATLAS SHRUGGED

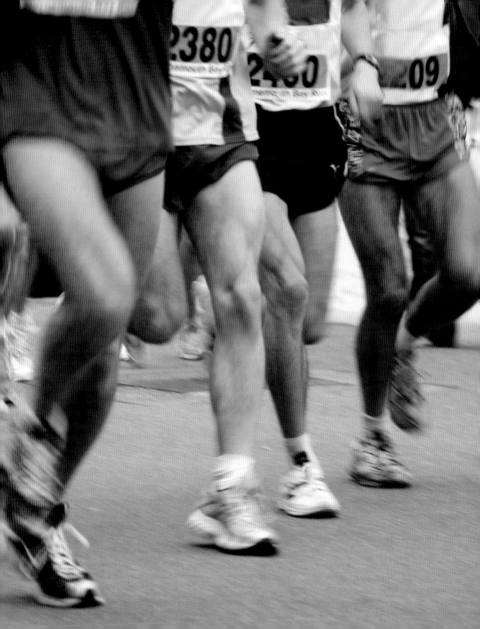

WEEK TWELVE: YOUR TRAINING PROGRAMME AND DIARY

		YOUR DAILY NOTES
MON	5 mins warm up, 5 mins slightly quicker jog, 5 mins cool down (total 15 mins). Keep relaxed throughout the session.	
TUE	Rest.	
WED	5 mins warm up, 15 mins easy jog, 5 mins cool down (total 25 mins). Keep walks at a moderate pace and don't push yourself on the run.	
THU	Rest. These next few rest days are crucial in preparing your body for race day so keep relaxed and as stress free as possible.	
FRI	Rest. Stretch to stay loose and think ahead to the race day.	
SAT	Your 5 km race or rest. Choose the day which suits you best.	
SUN	Your 5 km race or rest. Choose the day which suits you best.	

THIS WEEK

 DO – Enjoy yourself! This is what you have worked for so there is nothing to worry about.

 CONSIDER – Thinking about how the programme, and race went, and what you might challenge yourself with next.

 DON'T – Get disheartened if things don't go exactly to plan because you have made huge strides just to get this far.

REWARD

You've completed the challenge so you choose the reward!

Checklist

- ☐ Running shoes
- ☐ Socks
- ☐ Shorts or running pants
- ☐ T-shirt or vest
- ☐ Jacket or warm top
- ☐ Cap or peak
- ☐ Sunglasses
- ☐ Vaseline and plasters
- ☐ Water bottle or sports drink
- ☐ Energy bar
- ☐ Race number, safety pins and timing chip
- ☐ Map and transport details for getting to the start
- ☐ Towel and wet wipes

Try to get as much good sleep as you can this week as you may struggle to sleep well the night before the race because of excitement. When the night before the race does arrive, have a decent dinner but nothing too heavy, and avoid alcohol and caffeine (there will be plenty of time to celebrate afterwards!). Try to stick to your normal sleep routine, although you may need to go to bed a bit earlier if the morning start is an early one.

On the morning of the race have breakfast and a glass of water an hour (or more) before the race. Do not eat or drink anything you are not used to or you may upset your stomach. This is not the time to be experimenting! Then spend a couple of minutes running through the details of the race in your head for the final time.

Get to the start early so you can get your bearings and prepare yourself. If necessary, wear a warm top

6-10

If you need a performance boost in the day then a short sleep – or a power nap if you want to sound smart – of just six to 10 minutes could do the trick. If this sounds like something for you then keep the nap short and sharp so you avoid waking up feeling groggy. (22)

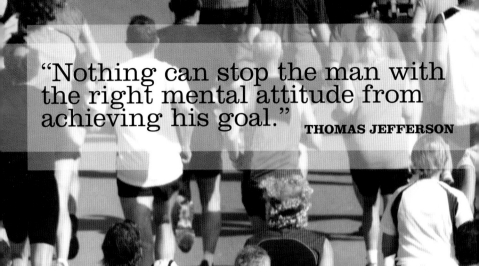

"Nothing can stop the man with the right mental attitude from achieving his goal." **THOMAS JEFFERSON**

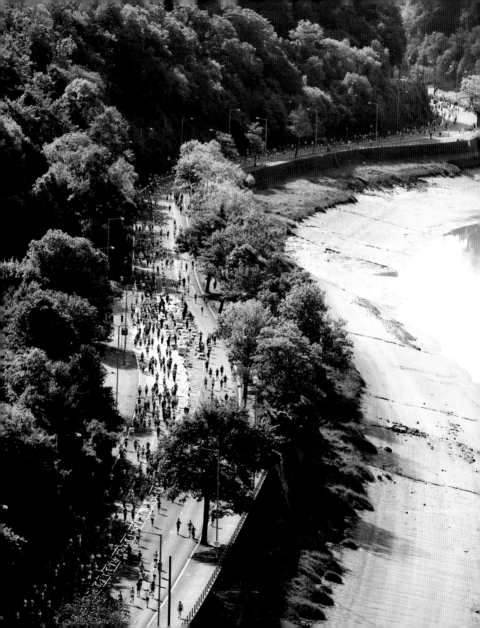

you can hand to a friend nearer the start time (or even an old one you don't mind throwing away). Many races will have a bag drop-off point where you can leave your belongings, which you collect when you have finished.

Up until now you have probably been running alone or with a friend, but running a race with a lot of other people is a very different, and may even be a little daunting. There is a buzz of anticipation at the start. Enjoy the atmosphere but don't get carried away and go charging off too fast. This is an easy thing to do so keep focused on your own race and do not worry about others around you. In particular do not let it concern you if it seems everyone is passing you – you are not trying to win the race.

In the bigger races with lots of runners it is likely that the course will get congested. Accept that this may slow you down and don't waste valuable energy weaving in and out of the other runners only to find yourself in the same situation a few metres further up the field. You will find yourself running more than 5 km if you start weaving so pick and choose carefully when to overtake. Keep an eye open for runners ahead of you slowing down or stopping suddenly. If you need to stop then gradually move to the edge of the field before you do so.

But finally, you are ready… enjoy your race!

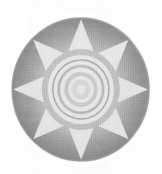

Have you ever noticed how refreshed and good you feel after exercising once the huffing and puffing has stopped?

Numerous studies have found there is a direct link between exercising and feeling happy and satisfied with your life. Getting a smile on your face – can there be a better reason for you to exercise? (23)

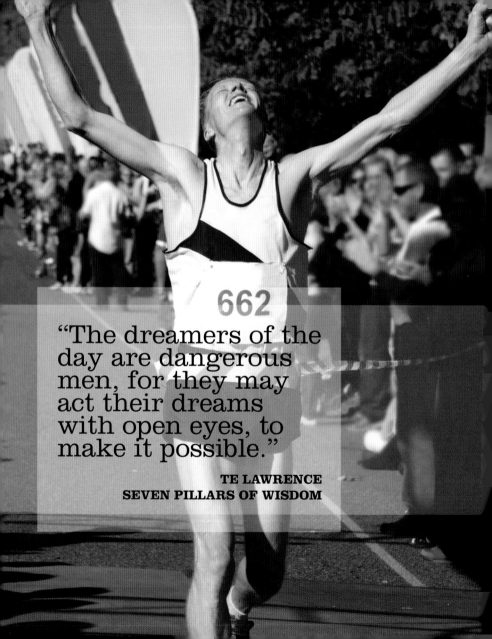

"The dreamers of the day are dangerous men, for they may act their dreams with open eyes, to make it possible."

TE LAWRENCE
SEVEN PILLARS OF WISDOM

that's it!

Week twelve completed

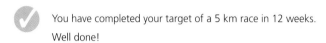 You have completed your target of a 5 km race in 12 weeks. Well done!

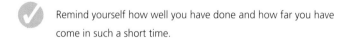 Remind yourself how well you have done and how far you have come in such a short time.

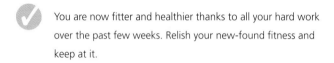 You are now fitter and healthier thanks to all your hard work over the past few weeks. Relish your new-found fitness and keep at it.

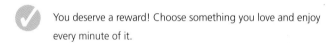 You deserve a reward! Choose something you love and enjoy every minute of it.

Your notes at the
end of the week

what now?

Now's the time to look ahead

So that's it then? A big sigh of relief at having completed your challenge. But now what...

You might have won your bet, lost some weight, got back into your favourite dress, whatever it was that inspired you 12 weeks ago to take up this challenge. So what happens next? Do you simply slink back and become the fittest pizza muncher in the area? Or do you keep up this new lifestyle?

You will probably be in one of two camps at this stage. You might be in the, "That's enough of that exercise stuff, I've proved to everyone I can do it so they can all shut up!" Or you might be in the super enthusiastic camp that thinks, "Right that was fun, what's the next challenge?"

If you are in the "Let's pack it in camp" that's fine, it's your choice. But it really would be a shame to waste all the hard work you've put in over the past few weeks. Nobody says you have to become a fitness fanatic because simply maintaining your recent level of exercise – a few days a week – is okay. Find a similar challenge to the one you have just completed

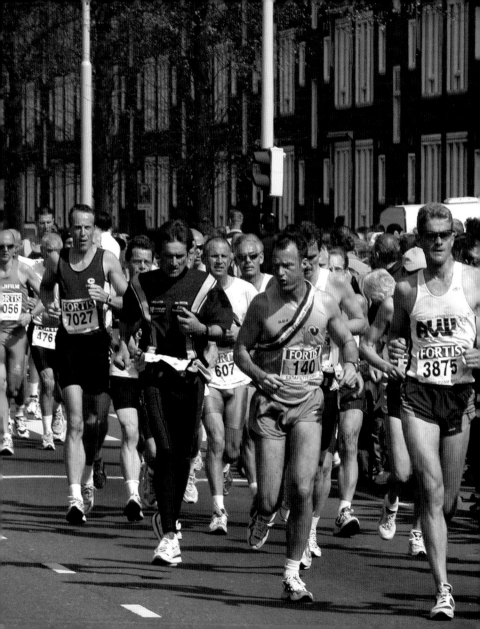

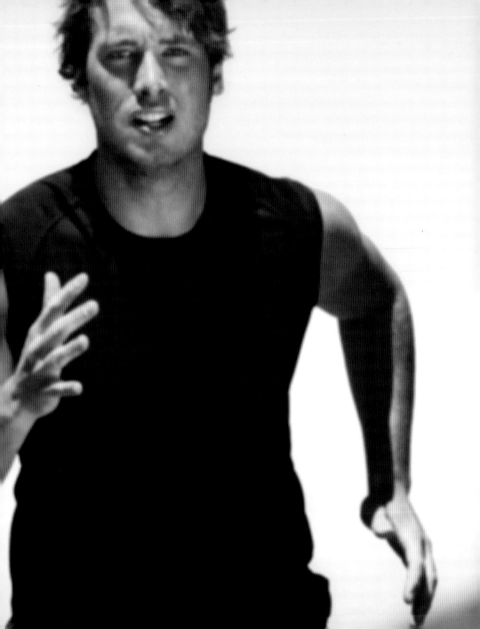

if that's what you need to inspire you, or mix it up and take up a new activity. There's no rule that says you have to only run. Spend some time swimming, cycling, or dancing – whatever it is that keeps you motivated and keeps you fit.

Spend a few moments thinking back over the highlights of the last few weeks and try to remember the journey you have taken. Read back over your notes as it will help to jog your memory. You have done all the tough groundwork already; keeping fit and healthy is a lot easier than getting there in the first place. By all means take a bit of a break but don't leave it too long as it is not difficult to slip back into old bad habits.

If you're in the super-enthusiastic camp then you'll need no such injection of new motivation. For you the world of fitness has probably opened up before you and you're wondering how you lived without it before. If you haven't already then start planning new challenges that will stretch you beyond the one you have just completed. Maybe now is the time to join a local running club and see how far you can take this?

A word of warning though: do not overstretch yourself and start doing too much. It is easy to get carried away and want to exercise every day but you have to remember that keeping fit and healthy has to slot in with the demands of your lifestyle. Over the last 12 weeks you have been training for a few days a week so make sure you can find the time for any extra sessions you may want to start doing. It is better to keep doing a few quality training sessions than attempt to do too much and fail. This can lead to frustration and ultimately you giving up.

Like those in the not-so-keen camp, consider taking up a different activity like swimming or cycling so as to keep your interest levels high. Keeping fit and healthy should be fun so don't be afraid to mix it up and change the things you do.

If you ever start to feel exercising is becoming a trudge then remind yourself of what inspired you to get going in the first place. Think back to successes you have had and the positive feelings you felt when getting fit.

Whatever route you decide to take from here, the last 12 weeks should have given you something very powerful to draw on. You now know you can decide on a challenge, plan the route, stick to the plan and get to the end successfully. It's something you can take forward in all areas of you life.

We hope you have enjoyed your journey so far. We wish you the best of luck going forward, whatever you decide is the next challenge for you!

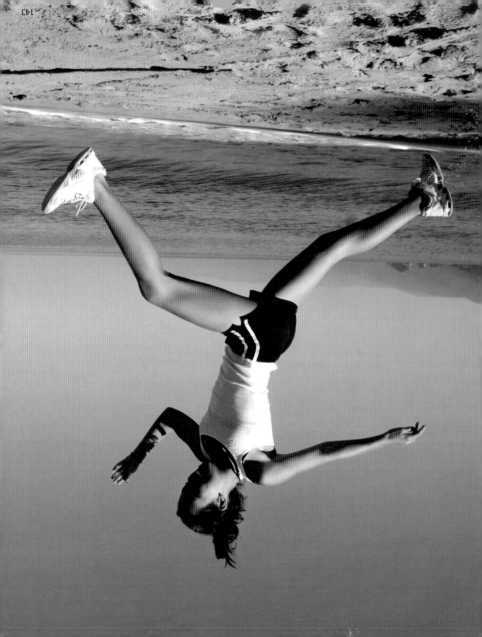

First published in 2013 by
New Holland Publishers (UK) Ltd
London • Cape Town • Sydney • Auckland
www.newhollandpublishers.com

A catalogue record for this book is available from the British Library.

ISBN 978 1 78009 233 1

This book has been produced for New Holland Publishers by
Chase My Snail Ltd
London • Cape Town
www.chasemysnail.com

Designer: Darren Exell
Photo Editor: Anthony Ernest
Consultant Sports Psychologist: Russell Murphy
Proof Readers: Daniel Rathbone, Timothy Shave, Hannah Shipman
Production: Marion Storz

2 4 6 8 10 9 7 5 3 1

Printed and bound in China by Toppan Leefung Printing Ltd.